T0202107

The Ethics
of Workplace Privacy

P.I.E.-Peter Lang

Bruxelles · Bern · Berlin · Frankfurt am Main · New York · Oxford · Wien

SALTSA
A Joint Programme for Working Life Research in Europe

SALTSA is a programme of partnership in European working life research run by the Swedish National Institute for Working Life (NIWL/ALI) and the Swedish Confederations of Trade Unions (LO), Professional Employees (TCO) and Professional Associations (SACO).

The aim of SALTSA is to generate applicable research results of a high academic standard and relevance. Research is largely project-based.

Research is carried out in three areas:
* the labour market
* work organisation
* the work environment

The Work Environment and Health Programme

Research on work environment and health focuses instruments and methods for healthier working conditions, the effects of certain risks in current working life as well as the conditions of selected groups of workers. Projects are designed with the ambition to contribute to the political debate and decision-making, applied occupational health and work environment management as well as participatory processes involving social partners in European working life.

Chairman of the SALTSA Programme is Professor Lars Magnusson and programme secretary for this area is Charlotta Krafft.

website: www.niwl.se/saltsa

Sven Ove HANSSON & Elin PALM (eds.)

The Ethics
of Workplace Privacy

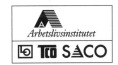

SALTSA — JOINT PROGRAMME
FOR WORKING LIFE RESEARCH IN EUROPE
The National Institute for Working Life and The Swedish Trade Unions in Co-operation

"Work & Society"
No.50

This book is the result of two interdisciplinary workshops on 'Workplace privacy' organised by the Philosophy Unit, Royal Institute of Technology, Stockholm, with the support of the Swedish National Institute for Working Life (NIWL) through the Joint Programme for Working Life Research in Europe (SALTSA).

© P.I.E.-PETER LANG S.A.
Presses Interuniversitaires Européennes
Brussels, 2005
1 avenue Maurice, 1050 Brussels, Belgium
info@peterlang.com; www.peterlang.net

ISSN 1376-0955
ISBN 90-5201-293-8
US ISBN 0-8204-6655-7
D/2005/5678/24
Printed in Germany

Bibliographic information published by "Die Deutsche Bibliothek"
"Die Deutsche Bibliothek" lists this publication in the "Deutsche Nationalbibliografie"; detailed bibliographic data is available in the Internet at <http://dnb.ddb.de>.

CIP available from the British Library, GB and the Library of Congress, USA.

Table of Contents

Preface

During the major part of the 20th century, there seemed to be a general tendency in the industrial world towards more humane workplaces. Health and safety regulations have contributed to safer workplaces, employer-employee relations have become less hierarchical and more conducive to personal development, and many factors have contributed to improve the social standing of employees. However, in the last few years we have seen developments that seem to go in the reverse direction. On some workplaces, workers find themselves controlled with computerised devices that allow for a more detailed monitoring than what ever has been possible before. Furthermore, biomedical tests are now available, that can provide employers with details about their employees that were unthinkable only a couple of decades before.

In recent academic work, there are two discourses on employee privacy. One of these deals with the effects of new genetic and biotechnological methods for screening and monitoring of workers' health. The other deals with the effects of surveillance technologies such as Closed Circuit Television (CCTV) and various methods for intercepting and analysing computer communications. The purpose of this collection of essays is to draw these two discussions together, in order to achieve a better understanding of the emerging total picture. Our emphasis is on ethical analysis and on the identification of policy options.

This book stems from an interdisciplinary cooperation on workplace privacy initiated by the SALTSA, a Swedish programme for working life research that is a joint undertaking by the National Institute for Working Life and the three Swedish confederations of employees LO, TCO, SACO. The book has grown out of discussions at our two workshops in Sigtuna, Sweden, in November 2002 and November 2003. We would like to thank the participants who have not written chapters in this book but who have contributed to the discussions leading up to this work. Thanks to: Elizabeth Ettorre, Kalle Grill, Lars Lindblom, David Mason, Martin Petersson and Charles Raab. Thanks are also due to SALTSA and in particular to Anders Schaerström and Charlotta Krafft.

We hope that the book will contribute to facilitate policy discussions and make concerned parties better prepared to make well-informed decisions on control, surveillance, and privacy on workplaces.

Stockholm, December 14, 2004

Sven Ove Hansson, Elin Palm

New Technologies – New Ethical Challenges

Sven Ove HANSSON and Elin PALM

Since the beginning of the industrial revolution, the automatisation of work has continuously been extended to new types of work tasks. One of the latest developments is the automatisation of surveillance. Some of the tasks previously conducted by foremen and supervisors can now be performed by various forms of Electronic Performance Monitoring (EPM) systems, that electronically collect, store and analyse employee performance. The methods used include telephone call accounting, keystroke and computer time tracking, location monitoring by smart cards and beepers, computer file monitoring, screen sharing capabilities on networks, and video camera observation. Furthermore, Radio Frequency IDs (RFID), Global Information Systems (GIS) and biometric verification systems can be used to identify employees' geographical location and to trace their movements. The employee's health status and capabilities can be monitored with biomedical tests such as genetic tests, pregnancy tests, and AIDS tests.

Arguably, each of the new surveillance and monitoring technologies has, *per se*, only limited effects on work life conditions. However, in combination they give rise to a new situation in which workers can be monitored and controlled to previously unknown degrees.

At least three reasons can be given why this new situation has only attracted relatively little attention. One such reason is that the very concept of privacy at work seems problematic. Whereas we expect a high degree of privacy in our homes and in some of the places where we spend our spare time, we traditionally expect a much lower degree of privacy in the workplace. The employee is expected to carry out certain tasks specified in her employment contract. As a part of the contract, the employer is entitled to a certain amount of insight in and control of her doings within the workplace. The question then is, what, if any, place is there for privacy?

A second reason is that we are accustomed to discuss privacy invasions in terms of governmental invasions in the private affairs of individuals. In that sense, our view of surveillance is still largely coloured by the Orwellian "Big Brother" dystopia in which central government is in charge of surveillance. This perception may obscure new patterns of surveillance in which individual companies rather than central government perform much of the monitoring.

The third reason is that biomedical testing and electronic surveillance have mostly been discussed as separate issues in isolation from each other, rather than as two aspects of the same phenomenon. As a consequence of this, their combined effects have not always been perceived.

The purpose of this book is to contribute to a more focused public and scholarly discussion on privacy intrusive practices on workplaces. The book is divided into three parts. The first of these parts introduces and analyses genetic testing on workplaces and the second electronic privacy invasions on workplaces. In the third part, ethical analyses are presented that approach the privacy invasions associated with both types of technology.

The first part, devoted to genetic technology, begins with a contribution by Gerard de Vries in which he urges us to appraise the potential of genetic technology realistically. The picture of genetic technology that emerges in public discussions is often based on unwarranted genetic determinism and unrealistic apprehensions about what genetic technology can accomplish. de Vries shows how the emerging practice of predictive medicine differs from clinical medicine in locating persons at risk rather than answering to the needs of persons with health complaints who take the initiative to contact a practitioner. The rise of predictive medicine has led to new power relations, and the patient is assigned a new role and new responsibilities. Occupational medicine is likely to adopt these new developments in the future. Therefore its role in relation to clinical and predictive medicine needs to be redefined.

Marja Sorsa and Karel Van Damme argue that since the scientific basis of the predictability of present genetic tests is thin, these tests should be treated with caution. They identify conditions under which genetic tests can be morally acceptable and argue that, most often, removal of hazardous agents and prevention of worker exposure should be the solution rather than the removal of sensitive workers who have been identified through genetic testing. They admit that there are cases in which genetic testing may be considered acceptable, but maintain that it should then be used for prevention rather than for prediction.

In the second part of the book, devoted to privacy relevant uses of information technology, the stage is set in a chapter by Simon Rogerson and Mary Prior. They identify and describe the major ways in which information and communication technologies (ICT) are used to monitor employees. Technology developers seldom pay sufficient attention to the actual or potential privacy intrusive implications of the technology, and many employers use surveillance capable technology without assessing whether such technology is necessary. In conclusion, they propose a model for social impact analysis that is intended to ensure that monitoring practices are socially and ethically acceptable.

In his contribution, Colin Bennett begins by reviewing the major policy approaches that have been taken to cope with privacy issues in different countries. Different mixtures of regulation, self-regulation, and technological instruments have been used to protect workers' privacy. In the latter part of the paper, he investigates the privacy aspects of increased workplace mobility. Mobile electronic equipment, in particular location-based services such as GPS make it possible to monitor the mobile worker. The traditional concept of the workplace as a geographically defined area is now outdated as for protecting privacy, and new regulatory approaches will have to be developed.

The third part of the book is devoted to ethical analysis. It begins with two chapters that provide analyses in terms of two concepts that are central to workplace ethics, namely privacy and discrimination.

Philip Brey provides an outline of the privacy discussion up till now and points to what he sees as lacking; an operationalised notion of privacy that suffices to distinguish between different types of private affairs, privacy rights, and privacy intrusions. He then uses his suggested operationalised notion to analyse workplace privacy in particular.

Sven Ove Hansson's chapter discusses genetic discrimination but also other forms of injustices and inequalities that may arise in workplaces due to surveillance and control practices. He concludes that protection of employees' privacy is often the best way to protect them against discrimination and other injustices.

The last two chapters provide tools for ethical assessment of surveillance capable technology. Anders Persson contributes a set of ethical criteria that can be used to assess under what conditions workplace surveillance can be morally justifiable. These criteria specify conditions under which it may be morally acceptable to subject employees to privacy intrusive practices. The application of the criteria is exemplified by medical and electronic surveillance.

Elin Palm presents a dimensional analysis that is developed as an instrument for assessing actual or potential monitoring devices and practices. She proposes seven dimensions for analysing the severity of privacy intrusions. These dimensions can be used to alleviate the negative effects of a surveillance capable technology in cases where the technology itself cannot be eliminated. It is suggested that in most practical cases, the negative implications may be reduced along one or more of these dimensions. Every reduction along one dimension is to be considered an improvement.

PART I

THE GENETIC REVOLUTION IN THE WORKPLACE

CHAPTER 1

Genetic Screening at Work

Risk and Responsibility
in the Era of Predictive Medicine

Gerard DE VRIES

1. Introduction

At first sight, genetic screening of workers and job-applicants for susceptibility to occupational diseases may seem a very good idea. After all, early warning of increased susceptibility to specific occupational hazards can prevent employees developing work-related diseases and may help to reduce the employers' budget for sick-pay. Closer consideration, however, soon reveals serious ethical, social and legal problems related to workers' rights as well as to the very real prospect of discrimination and new kinds of inequality arising. Moreover, there are technical limitations to genetic screening at work. In fact, the potential for selecting workers and applicants on the basis of genetic traits is very limited indeed. Current tests have limited sensitivity and specificity. As a result of this, the level of both false negatives and false positives is high. Of course, sensitivity and specificity of tests may be expected to rise in the years to come. However, basic epidemiological science teaches us that, for rare diseases, decision-making based on screening will always remain an imprecise science, because even the smallest error in the sensitivity and/or specificity of the test will seriously reduce the accuracy of predictions (Van Damme and Castelyn, 2002).

In the past two decades, remarkable successes have been achieved in clinical genetics. However, it would be a mistake to extrapolate these successes to genetic screening at work. In the first place, the achievements in clinical genetics relate to diseases in which one or only a small number of genetic mutations are sufficient to cause disease. Genetic traits concerning work-related diseases, such as cancer and allergies, will, most likely, involve many genes, the many ways in which they interact, and their interactions with the environment. To make predictions about polygenetic diseases is of a fundamentally different nature from making predictions about monogenetic diseases. Secondly, genetic testing outside the context of families with known histories of a disease and without the possibility to also extensively test members of the family in question, requires different methodologies and is a qualitatively different task than studies currently undertaken in clinical genetics. A commission advising the UK government rightly concluded in July 1999 that "it will take major developments both in our understanding of common diseases and in genetic testing itself before genetic testing becomes a serious issue for employment practice" (Human Genetics Advisory Commission, 1999).

Large-scale use of genetic technologies to test workers and job-applicants is not to be expected in the short term. To conclude that public discussion about this issue is misplaced, ill-timed or unnecessary would, however, be mistaken. In the first place, technological developments, *e.g.* the introduction of low-cost DNA micro assays which can be used to screen for hundreds of genetic traits simultaneously to assess a person's special susceptibility to work place hazards, may rapidly change the situation. Secondly, the illusion that genetic technologies deliver accurate long-term predictions concerning the future state of health of individuals may lead to the temptation to use statistical genetic information for actuarial prediction purposes proving irresistible for many employers. The ethical, social and legal problems of genetic testing in work-related contexts only increase when this practice is based on unreliable technologies and illusions on the part of management.

Public discussion regarding genetic testing should therefore continue. However, current discussions are often misdirected on three points. Discussions are often based on unrealistic claims as to the predictive power of tests. This is particularly true of much comment in the media. Secondly, the starting point for much debate is the mistaken idea that technologies work as advertised. And finally, by taking a short-sighted focus on technologies, commentators tend to detract attention from related, wider developments in medicine and health care.

In this paper, I will first elaborate on these observations. The main thrust of the paper, however, is to argue that genetics-based medical diagnosis will accelerate and deepen a transformation in medical thinking that has already been developing for several decades. This transformation triggers a redistribution of responsibilities for health and disease. I will argue that the prime issue in the public debate about genetics should be this transformation and its consequences.

2. Public Discussions about Genetics

Recent developments in genetics have provoked a wide range of conflicting public reactions.

For many, genetics holds the promise of medicine preventing disease, rather than merely reacting to the onset of illness. Diagnostic tests to detect a genetic predisposition to certain conditions are already available. These include Huntington's disease, cystic fibrosis, Tay-Sachs disease, familial hypercholesterolemia and certain forms of breast cancer. More tests are expected to become available in the near future. These tests carry the promise of early diagnosis and – in most cases – also the promise of reducing the chances of developing the disease or making it easier to bear, as early treatment in the form of long-term medication or other forms of medical intervention, *e.g.* preventive operations, diets, or lifestyle-changes, can start long before symptoms appear. Effective tests for genetic traits related to the "big killer" diseases, like cancer and cardiovascular diseases, both of which involve many genes, those genes' interactions among themselves, and their interactions with the environment, are still a long way off. In fact, nobody knows whether this distant goal will ever be reached.

Genetics confronts society with serious social and ethical problems. Genetic diagnostics may present unimaginable dilemmas for individuals, *e.g.* in the case of genetic predisposition to breast cancer, whether or not to have bilateral mastectomy to reduce the chance of developing the disease in the long term. Those who have had genetic diagnostic tests may also have to face serious problems in the domains of insurance, employment and privacy. More far-reaching objections include the thesis that genetic tests used for prenatal diagnosis (leading to abortion, when genetic anomalies are discovered) or for the purpose of embryo-selection (pre-implantation diagnostics, PID), open the road to new forms of eugenics (Habermas, 2001).

The picture of genetics that emerges in the media is often based on wildly overstated claims and on unwarranted genetic deterministic ideas. Both the proponents of the new technology and their critics have to share the blame for this. Researchers in genetics in search of research grants often think that a little publicity cannot hurt and thus tend to exaggerate the potential usefulness of their work. What better reason for taxpayers to contribute to expensive research than the prospect of helping to prevent cancer, cardiac disease or Alzheimer's? Biotechnology companies join in. Having invested heavily in developing new genetic tests, the industry obviously has an interest in ensuring that their products are widely adopted. For this purpose, companies paint an overoptimistic picture of their products' potential. Interestingly enough, many critics who point to possible negative effects of genetic technologies accept the overstated claims made by scientists and the industry for their products at face value. The effect is that in the public domain, discussion is often based on exaggerated claims about the potential of genetics and the time required to achieve the promised results.

The reality of genetics research is less amenable to flamboyant claims. In the first place, the road from basic research to medical applications is long and tortuous. In the case of genetic diagnostics and screening a number of basic biological and statistical facts get in the way of quick and easy success. Genes offer only potentials, rather than a view on the individual that will eventually develop. The relation of genetic characteristics to physical and mental outcomes is, in most cases, purely statistical. Between genotype and phenotype numerous variables interfere in complex, and, as yet – and possibly forever – unpredictable ways. Except for a very small number of traits, virtually all the details of the processes through which phenotypes emerge are unknown. Nobody knows whether the distant goal of effective genetic tests for the polygenetic 'big killer' diseases will ever be achieved. Moreover, epidemiological arguments show that diagnostics outside the context of families with known histories of a disease, *e.g.* unsolicited population screening and genetic screening in the workplace, is of limited value.

A second factor frustrating the debate about genetics is an oversimplistic view of what the development and implementation of new technologies mean. In many discussions, genetic technology is presented as a monolith, and society, as its passive receiver, is cast as having only one choice: to either accept or reject the technology. Historical and social studies of technology show this picture to be utterly inadequate. Technologies not only change social practices, but in the process of their implementation, they themselves also take on new shapes. In the social shaping of technologies, many actors – including end-users, *i.e.* citizens – play roles. Successful implementation of technology often requires explicit regulation, and changes in attitudes and behaviour of those involved. Technologies do not make their appearance on an empty stage, but have to be imbedded in existing social structures. Technological determinism is a doctrine that is every bit as unfounded as genetic determinism.

To make an educated guess about the ways in which genetics will affect society, we therefore have to turn our attention not only to the potentials of the new technologies, but also to the contexts in which the new technologies emerge and will be implemented. To discuss seriously the impact of genetics on society we must therefore first understand medicine in its present state as a social practice.

Physicians of the 21st century will most likely spend an increasingly large portion of their time counselling patients on how to stay healthy. However, although the availability of genetic diagnostics and screening will help to advance this trend, it is first and foremost an effect of medical practitioners having already come to accept a new way of thinking, and working in practices that are organised around new principles. The soil in which genetic technologies will take root, has thus already been prepared by developments in medicine that are unrelated to genetics. Even if genetics did not take off, medicine in the 21st century would nonetheless have a different face from that which it has had for most of the 20th century.

Current interest in genetics is part of a transformation in medical science that has been under way for decades. This transformation can be characterised as a move from clinical, complaints-bound medicine to predictive, risk-oriented medicine. Modern epidemiology, health promotion and education, along with prenatal diagnostics – new branches on the tree of medicine – dating largely from the 1960s, 1970s and 1980s, were the earlier manifestations of a movement that is now boosted by genetics. Each of these areas has contributed to a new kind of thinking in medical science that defines problems of health and disease increasingly as problems of risks, and which draws primary attention to prevention, rather than cure, while distinguishing itself from earlier prevention-oriented public health efforts by its focus on the health of individuals, rather than communities.

3. Classical and Clinical Medicine

To better understand the context in which genetics will develop, and to get a view of the specific features of predictive medicine, it is necessary to analyse a number of features of health care systems in industrial societies. The purpose of this analysis is not to discover something that is hidden from view, but rather to highlight features we fail to notice because they are so close, so intimately linked to every day practices, that we take them for granted, allowing them to fall below our perception threshold. We have to distance ourselves from what has become too obvious to us. A brief historical digression may help in this regard.

The core ideas that have guided medical practice in the 20th century emerged in the 19th. In the early decades of that century, new ideas about medical knowledge and a new understanding of disease, new relations between doctors and patients, new attitudes towards the human

21

body and, eventually, new forms of power materialised (Foucault, 1975; Porter and Porter, 1989). 'Classical' medicine gave way to 'clinical medicine'. This change involved a complex interplay of institutions, practices and ideas.

Pre-1800 'classical medicine' conceived disease as a distinct onto-logical entity that did not depend on the particular body in which it might find itself. Within the patient's body, disease was thought to be able to circulate freely from one site to another with no essential altera-tion. The way a disease unfolded over time, rather than its spatial local-isation in the individual's body, was taken to be its main characteristic. In contrast, in 'clinical medicine' disease relates to the pathological condition of a specific internal organ. In 'clinical medicine', disease is specifically located in the body. As we will see, this seemingly abstract difference in concepts of disease has important practical consequences.

For physicians of the classical age, the starting-point of diagnosis was the patient's oral account of his suffering and other signs of sick-ness that he presented. To understand the disease, the doctor had to classify it on the basis of these signs and his knowledge about the natural course of diseases. Given the conception of disease of this period, there was hardly any need to inspect carefully the patient's body, nor its internal organs, simply because the disease might have taken root anywhere. Close examination of the patient's body was simply meaning-less. That doctors of the classical age seldom asked their patients to undress was therefore not out of prudishness. Similarly, as regards therapy, invasive action would mostly be misdirected. A doctor might try to ease suffering, *e.g.* by bloodletting, but his main advice consisted in prescribing rest, preferably at home. Hospitals were still asylums for the very poor and few recovered in these institutions. The most impor-tant thing was to let the disease take its natural course. Typical of classi-cal medicine is the message of the doctor which we may find in many 18th- and 19th-century novels, that the patient, having come through the 'crisis' of pneumonia and having survived the critical stage in the natu-ral course of the disease, will live.

All of this changed when, in the early 19th century, a new medical consciousness emerged and a new, clinical, conception of disease gained favour. Disease was no longer understood as a bundle of charac-ters disseminated throughout the body. It came to be conceptualised as the effect of pathological states of specific internal organs. The body itself had become ill. The physical examination, and the inspection of internal organs, therefore became the main diagnostic techniques. Instruments like the stethoscope and later, X-rays and other techniques to visualise the internal state of the body, and laboratory analyses of samples of blood, urine and tissues, helped to inform the doctor about the condition of specific organs and thus to identify the disease the patient was suffering from. The doctor's relationship with his/her patient changed dramatically because of this new approach. From someone who made a diagnosis mainly on the basis of the patient's accounts of their suffering, the physician had turned into a professional who had to ask his patient to undress to inspect his body, and even to use aggressive, invasive diagnostic and therapeutic techniques.

This transformation in the concept of disease not only affected the relationship between doctors and patients, but also had institutional consequences. In clinical medicine, laboratory analyses are important diagnostic instruments; in classical medicine, the laboratory played no role at all. The way hospitals are organised changed too. Patients came to be sorted into wards on the basis of their disease (with specialised wards for respiratory medicine, neurology, internal medicine, *etc.*), allowing comparison and thus facilitating a better understanding of the disease.

Wider consequences soon followed. Since the new clinical medical examination involved touching of naked bodies and invasive diagnostics, state authorities in the 19th century recognised that explicit rules were required to determine who can legitimately claim the authority for such privacy-invading actions. Who is allowed to ask patients to undress, to inspect bodies, to use invasive diagnostic techniques and therapies, to study corpses? Turning the medical world into an access-controlled profession, 19th-century laws on medical practice provided an answer to these questions. Permission to practise medicine was explicitly restricted by law. In the course of the century that followed, regulations have continuously been extended. Today, distribution of medical information is governed by laws on medical confidentiality, guaranteeing the patient that he can freely talk about his complaints with his doctor. Separate laws cover population screening and occupational medicine. After the Second World War it was recognised that the existing system of laws and regulations was not sufficient to prevent individuals from becoming the subject of unacceptable practices (such as medical experiments without consent which might have undermined trust in clinical medicine as a whole) and as a result, additional measures were put in place. Today, in most countries, the power of the medical profession is balanced by the principle of informed consent which requires the patient's explicit permission for all invasive medical diagnostic and therapeutic interventions. The distribution of responsibilities between doctors and patients that comes with clinical medicine is to a large extent explicitly prescribed by law.

The effects of these laws are two-fold: they put constraints on medical practice, but also allow the practitioner to practise. Licensing the medical profession protects individuals against quacks who may take advantage of their weak position and who may endanger their health. Regulation of doctor-patient relations and privacy provides protection for the individual in the social space of the surgery where he meets his physician; equally, regulations on occupational law protect employees. However, laws on medical practice also guide behaviour, not only of doctors, but also of their patients. Modern patients know what is expected when they enter a physician's office. They know that they may be asked to undress and to allow the doctor to perform invasive, and even painful, diagnostic actions. When the doctor has come to the conclusion that the patient is seriously ill and needs treatment, the patient knows he is expected to comply – to swallow prescribed pills, stay in bed, accept hospitalisation. By setting up a space in which intimacy and privacy may *legitimately* be invaded by doctors, the laws that regulate medicine make modern medicine possible. To illustrate the point, just imagine patients refusing to give their permission for physicians to inspect their bodies and instead, inviting them – in the manner of our 18th-century predecessors – to diagnose solely on the basis of their own descriptions of their suffering. Modern medicine would come to an abrupt end.

Regulations in social security have similar two-fold effects. In European welfare states, patients may be excused from the obligation to go to work. In what sociologists have called the 'sick role', the patient is allowed to withdraw from daily responsibilities and social obligations. Their only obligation is to do everything that may help to improve their health. Again, laws regulating the sick role have double effects. They protect the individual from the social disaster that would otherwise befall him in the event of incapacity to work and social services from individuals who might want to take unfair advantage of the social security safety net. However, they also put the patient under medical surveillance and open the social space necessary for intensive medical treatment. Physicians would obviously be at a loss if they had to treat patients in their offices while continuing their work, rather than in well-equipped hospitals.

Medicine, we may conclude from this short digression into the origins and the basis of 'clinical medicine', is a complex system which involves ideas, techniques, institutions and daily practices. Medicine also comes with specific distributions of responsibilities between physicians, patients and society at large that are partly explicitly laid down in law, and partly based on custom. To analyse this complex system, we have to recognise how it is constituted by a large number of mutually dependent conditions. Clinical medicine's ideas about the nature of disease would soon evaporate without a medical practice in which they could be successfully applied. That practice is enabled by a web of regulations which emerged when the concept of disease changed and a new configuration of the patient's body, of medical knowledge and of professional intervention constituted a power relation that called for regulation. Removal of one of these conditions will lead to a collapse of the health care system as a whole.

It would be futile to think that we can easily separate causes from effects in this complex web of relations. However, that is not necessary for our purpose. To discuss the impact of genetic diagnostics and screening, it will suffice to be aware that the new ideas and technologies that are currently becoming available will become embedded in a medical system that is constituted by many more elements than is usually acknowledged in current discussions on the impact of genetics.

4. Predictive Medicine

As health care systems of the 20th century are based on 'clinical medicine', we tend to take its practice, its institutions and conception of disease for granted. However, in the second half of the 20th century the nature of medicine gradually started to change. To illustrate this change, we may shortly review the ways in which research on Alzheimer's disease has been reported in the medical press.

In 1907, in a celebrated paper, Alzheimer presented a 51-year-old woman who suffered from jealous delusions, memory disturbances, disorientation, delirious episodes and hallucinations. Her state continued to worsen, up to the point where she spent her days in bed in a state of complete apathy and incontinence. A *post mortem* examination of her brain showed her brain tissues to have changed in previously unknown ways (Alzheimer, 1987). Alzheimer's work clearly represents 'clinical medicine' in Foucault's sense. Whereas early 19th-century physicians would consider the woman to be 'possessed' by an illness, the aim of Alzheimer's examination was to identify the disorder by locating its causes in the body (*i.e.* in the patient's brain tissues).

For the sake of contrast, we may take a look at an issue of the *Journal of the American Medical Association* that reviewed progress in work on Alzheimer's disease 90 years after its discovery (Morison-Bogorod, 1997). As in the past, an important part of research is located in the laboratory, where the focus of attention has shifted from brain tissues to genes and molecules. However, what distinguishes contemporary work from the efforts of Alzheimer, is not this shift nor the increased sophistication of laboratory equipment that comes with it. More important is a change in the aim of research. Current research in Alzheimer's disease no longer focuses exclusively on the causes of disease and therapeutic options. Identifying those who are at risk of developing Alzheimer's disease, long before symptoms of the disease present themselves, has become a major goal in itself. Research is therefore also conducted on people who complain of no illness, *i.e.* subjects who, according to the criteria of clinical medicine, are in good health. Important advances are foreseen for the near future. Both genetics and epidemiological studies are reported to have contributed significantly to the task of identifying people and even ethnic groups who are at risk of developing Alzheimer disease. These studies are expected to lay the foundations for new health education and screening programs.

This example illustrates how the rise of 'predictive medicine' has consequences on various levels covered in the discussion of clinical medicine above, *i.e.* the nature of medical knowledge, the institutions of medicine and the nature of diagnostic practice and the doctor – patient relationship. As we will see, regulation of new medical practices has so far lagged behind developments in medicine. Because of this delay, the distribution of responsibilities in predictive medicine has taken a specific, and in some respects, troublesome turn.

With the rise of predictive medicine, health care has taken on a new shape. In the first place, we observe that both medical epistemology and the concept of 'disease' have changed. Knowledge about health risks is essentially statistical in nature; statements about risks are propositions about the probability of adverse events. The probabilistic nature of risk represents not just a matter of insufficient knowledge, but reflects objective constraints on what is knowable. This is not only true for lifestyle-induced risks, but also for genetic risks. The change in epistemology is reflected in definitions of disease that are discussed in the scientific press. In clinical medicine, disease was defined as a type of internal state of the body, which is either an impairment of normal functional ability, or a reduction of one or more functional abilities caused by environmental agents. A recent proposal for a definition of 'disease' however reads: "disease is a state that places individuals at increased risk of adverse consequences" (Temple *et al.*, 2001). In predictive medicine, disease has become an intrinsically probabilistic concept. Uncertainty is no longer attributed to the acknowledged imperfections of current knowledge (upholding the ideal of achieving certainty about deterministic physiological processes), but rather has moved to the object of medical science. The change in epistemology is reflected in a transformation of the object of medical knowledge. Statistical knowledge refers to populations, rather than to individuals. The social scale of medical knowledge is therefore extended. As the concepts of predictive risk-oriented medicine refer to populations that also include people who – in the clinical view – are healthy, *i.e. not yet* ill, also the timescale of the concept of 'disease' is extended. When 'risk' is used to depict the state of an individual's health, the individual is located in a population that is extended both in time and social space.

The concept of risk thus blurs the distinction between (individual) health and disease that was fundamental to clinical medicine. Someone who is found to be 'at risk' of developing a serious disease in the years or perhaps decades ahead, is not ill in the clinical meaning of the term. This has important social consequences. Simply being deemed to be 'at risk' does not give a right to appeal to current laws that regulate for sickness in welfare states. Employers expect their 'at-risk' employees to report dutifully at his work to do his job. Insurance companies, however, may take another view. The fact that someone has tested positive for a risk and knows the outcome of the test may be a reason to exclude him from insurance, to ask for a higher premium, or to shorten the term of the insurance contract. Although clinically speaking not ill, for the insurance company's purposes the policy-holder is not healthy either. Employers may take a similar view of job-applicants.

In the second place, the example of the changes in medicine's approach to Alzheimer's disease also shows how medicine moves into new social spaces and starts to involve new institutions. From the clinical setting, *i.e.* the physical examination of the patient in the doctor's surgery and the examination of blood, urine and tissues in a laboratory, the medical forum shifts to extended networks that include epidemiological data banks, laboratories, research institutes, and programs for health education. Predictive medicine requires co-operation between clinicians and pathologists with a large number of professionals, within and without the traditional medical field: epidemiologists, geneticists, but also psychologists, sociologists, health educators, and social workers. The distinction between medical and non-medical actors thus becomes opaque and laws concerning medical confidentiality and the privacy of medical data need to be reviewed. Neither psychologists who counsel patients in a centre for clinical genetics, nor communication experts who help to set up health education programs, are usually licensed medical doctors. Nevertheless, their work is essential to predictive medicine. Responsibilities are redistributed and may become unclear. In some cases, especially in genetics, the patient's active involvement is required to locate members of his family and to convince them that they also need to be tested, as a full picture of the genetic make-up and disease history of relatives is necessary before the results can be considered significant. What does this imply for the responsibility for making a diagnosis? Who has failed if a genetic test cannot be completed because a patient did not succeed in convincing his relatives to co-operate?

Turning, finally, to the nature of medical practice and to the doctor-patient relationship, we may observe that although, as is typically the case in clinical medicine, the initiative for a medical consultation may still be taken by the individual (who wants to have an assessment of his future health or the health of his offspring), the consultation may, equally, be prompted by a government institution, an employer, or a research institute. This changes the nature of the medical intervention. In many cases, in genetics medical diagnosis will require limited invasive action. The subject may be asked to provide a blood sample and to answer a questionnaire. However, in a different sense the subject has to expose himself. To bee designated 'at risk' implies being located within a network of factors drawn from observations of others, *i.e.* to be designated as part of a 'risk group'. In many cases, this network of factors is embodied in an abstract form, in databanks and theories of epidemiology. In some cases, however, it may have a more familiar face. In the case of genetic diseases, the person 'at risk' becomes someone who shares a fate with his relatives. In many cases, he will find himself have to seek their co-operation to achieve a significant risk assessment. Troubled family relations may have to be re-established. The difference between 'being family' in a biological and a social sense becomes manifest. Birthday parties and other family get-togethers may suddenly take on a whole new character.

5. Risk and Responsibility

The rise of predictive medicine not only implies the introduction of new diagnostic instruments, theories of disease and a promise of early diagnosis and reducing chances of developing a disease by taking counter-measures long before the disease manifests itself. Predictive medicine also comes with a re-distribution of responsibilities related to disease.

As a rule, in the clinical setting there is little doubt about the nature of medical action, about the question of who is responsible for taking action, nor about whose body will be the subject of the action. In the clinical setting, medical power has a recognisable face. An extensive system of laws and regulations helps to balance this power and to protect the patient. All of this changes when one moves to the field of predictive medicine.

Individuals who enter the area of predictive medicine will not immediately notice this difference. The institutes they have to go to are, in many cases, the same as they were used to visit to access clinical care. The physicians they meet will not have put their white coats away when a visitor comes for a consultation about health risks, rather than for treatment for a physical or a mental complaint. Those seeking to access predictive medicine will soon find themselves facing a strikingly different social situation to that which they may previously have known. The institutions they will have to relate to are organised in complex networks and include not only traditional medical professionals, but also members of professions which are outside what would have traditionally been regarded as the medical world. The distribution of responsibilities is complex, if not opaque. Laws to regulate and balance the power of this new complex have either yet to be introduced or are derived from regulations originally grafted onto clinical medicine, and thus lack the detailed regulations necessary for predictive medicine. A functional equivalent for the regulation of the 'sick role' to help protect those who are 'at risk' from adverse social consequences has yet not been introduced. As we will see, the effect of laws and regulations in predictive medicine lagging behind medical practice is that, at the end of the day, it is the 'at risk' individual who has to bear the burden of the responsibilities ensuing from his status.

Let us suppose an individual has consulted an institute for predictive medicine. He meets his doctor (a family doctor, a clinical geneticist, or a doctor in occupational medicine) who has told him that he has been found to be at risk of developing a serious disorder. What does this actually mean? To answer that question, it is helpful to review briefly the history of the concept of risk as several layers of meaning have come to be superimposed on the concept of 'health risk'.

The first meaning of 'risk' was roughly equivalent to 'danger'. The first attested examples of this usage date from 16th-century Italy. The word was used in nautical contexts, especially in the context of trips to the Indies.

In the 18th century, 'risk' came to have a new and more precise meaning. It was introduced in the theory of games of chance and acquired the meaning of what in contemporary probability theory is called 'mean-' or 'expected value', *i.e.* the product of the probability that an event will happen and the value of its outcome. In the 18th century, 'risk' was still used for both negative and positive outcomes. Later on, the concept was to be used to refer solely to adverse events.

29

The technical meaning of the concept of risk introduced in the 18th century is still in use, for example in the context of risk analyses of technical installations, *e.g.* nuclear power plants. Such analyses study trees of events in which a succession of little accidents with known frequencies of incidence trigger a major event, *e.g.* the meltdown of the reactor. The idea of risk analysis is to calculate the expected value of a major event on the basis of the probabilities of interacting smaller events, and to use this value, for example, to compare the 'risk' of nuclear energy with the risk of other energy sources.

The concept has also been in use in economics since the 1920s, in particular in investment theory. Whereas risk analyses of engineers focus on trees of events, economic risk analysis focuses on decision-trees. Today's business schools train future managers to use these methods to evaluate their decisions: which parts of the company or a stock-portfolio have to be closed or sold given the probability that they will produce losses that may endanger the company as a whole? While the mathematics of risk analysis in economics is similar to the mathematics of technical risk analysis, the perspective and the concept of probability that are used are different. Economic risk assessment is based on the so-called 'subjective' or Bayesian concept of probability, rather than the 'objective' (relative frequency) concept of probability that is used in engineering.

Medical use of the term 'risk' has yet another background. It was introduced in grand scale epidemiological studies of cardiovascular diseases and the relationship between smoking and lung cancer, conducted in the 1950s and 1960s. In this context, 'risk' refers to empirical probabilities based on population studies, *i.e.* to relative frequencies (rather than expected value) – for example, the probability that someone will get lung cancer after having smoked heavily for 25 years. However, from the 1970s, 'risk' has also been used in medicine in the decision-theoretical sense of the term, as in economics. For example, to choose between alternative courses of treatment, a physician may try to assess the options in terms of the overall risks they present to the patient. Medical decision theory based on Bayesian statistics has become an expanding discipline over the last forty years.

Lastly, consider the way 'risk' is dealt with in legal contexts. To consciously expose somebody to the risk of damage, *i.e.* to consciously take a risk, may in some cases be a reason for a conviction or liability for a damage-claim. For example, in a famous ruling, the Dutch High Court convicted someone who had sent a poisoned cake to kill a relative for homicide, although the postman delivered the cake on the wrong address where it killed an unknown stranger. By using the post service to deliver the poisoned cake, the person had consciously taken a risk, for which he was committed.

So what is communicated when somebody is told by his doctor that, because of his lifestyle, work environment or genetic disposition, he is at risk for developing a serious disease in the future? Different layers of meaning become activated. While the doctor may say: "You are at risk for developing a serious disorder," what this actually means is: "The relative frequency of developing this disorder in groups of people with whom you share certain characteristics, has been found to be higher than in groups of people who are similar to you in many respects, but who lack these characteristics." It may also mean: "It is known that people who carry this mutation have a higher chance of developing this disorder than people who don't have this mutation. The specific mechanism may be as yet unknown, but we have good reason to believe that there is a chance that the mutation triggers processes that will do damage to your health." These may be the doctor's words, but what his patient is more likely to understand is: "You are in serious danger!"

In the follow-up of the doctor's communication, new layers of the concept of risk are activated. The consultation will typically focus on the options available to lower the risk: a change in life-style, a job-change, a diet, medication, a preventive operation, perhaps. Thus the patient is invited to look at his own life in the way a manager looks at his company. Whereas a business-manager may have to consider the painful decision to close down a department – causing loss of work and social insecurity for many – a woman at risk of breast cancer may be placed in a similar, but even more painful dilemma: is preventive amputation of her breasts necessary to reduce the chance of the deadly disease developing in the decades ahead?

In the case of a genetic disease, the follow-up may also take another turn. The question has to be discussed whether the risk impacts on offspring. Should the patient abstain from having biological children of his own? Should a pregnancy that has already started be terminated? Future parents are asked to look at their relationship with their children as if they were judges who being asked to decide a case in which they have the most direct interest. Are they to be held responsible for the damage they may cause to their offspring, if they consciously decide to take the risk to have their own biological children (rather than adopting a child), or to continue a pregnancy that has already started?

The fact that is communicated ("relative frequency," "a mutation's probability to trigger adverse consequences") and the message that is received ("you are in serious danger") thus lead to new roles and responsibilities for the subject at risk, *i.e.*, the role of the manager of his own life, and/or that of a judge, forced to decide crucial questions about his relationship with his offspring. And all of this is prompted by the word "risk."

So, although there are many similarities between the position of a patient in clinical medicine and the position of someone who is at risk, there are also major differences.

In the first place, the powers that a patient in clinical medicine has to face are known, well-defined and regulated by law. As discussed above, the situation in predictive medicine is more complicated and opaque. Moreover, whereas in clinical medicine the sick person can withdraw from social life and is excused from many responsibilities, in predictive medicine, the person at risk is assigned new and sometimes heavy responsibilities – he may even have to perform as a kind a manager or a judge over his body and life. And whereas the welfare state's regulations of the sick role protect the individual from social disaster, current laws as yet provide no such security for those who are found to be at risk. In fact, the person at risk may find his options in accessing insurance cover to be significantly reduced.

Individuals do not have to carry the burden that comes with being found to be at risk alone. Various experts, including psychologists and social workers, are ready to assist in dealing with the new dilemmas posed and to help individuals to learn how to interpret and balance difficult, statistical information. Patient groups are available to meet others who happen to find themselves in a similar situation. But at the end of the day, the individual, and the individual alone has to decide what should be done. In clinical genetics the principle of autonomy has been rigorously adopted as a guiding principle: genetic experts may advise, but in the end, the decision about what is to be done is up to the individual patient. In this we see the legacy of post-World War II clinical medicine. As opposed to judges and managers, however, few are adequately prepared for this task. Neither are these choices necessarily made within a generous timeframe: decisions about terminating a pregnancy, for example, sometimes have to be made within weeks, if not days.

6. Health Care in the Risk Society

Few who contact a doctor or a centre for clinical genetics for a risk assessment will be aware of the new responsibilities they will have to face. The institutions they visit are, in many respects, identical to ordinary hospitals. But in the weeks or months that follow, the differences will become clear. Some may come to think that 'if they had known all of this' they would not have taken this road. However, meanwhile, the family may already have become involved, and the perspective of life-management may have been internalised. All the while, the first message, 'you are in danger', is at the forefront of their minds.

Why do we take the shift of responsibility that comes with predictive medicine for granted, or even welcome the idea that people have a responsibility for their future health as a sign of emancipation?

Charles Dickens' novel *Hard Times*, published in 1854, contains a dialogue that can easily be translated to contemporary situations. When Louisa Gradgrind, the daughter of the notorious Mr. Gradgrind, experiences doubts about her forthcoming marriage and sighs '*Father, I have often thought that life is very short,*' her father answers:

'*It is short, no doubt, my dear. Still, the average duration of human life is proved to have increased of late years. The calculations of various life assurance and annuity offices, among other figures which cannot go wrong, have established that fact.*'

'*I speak of my own life, Father.*'

'*Oh indeed? Still,*' said Mr. Gradgrind, '*I need not point out to you, Louisa, that it is governed by the laws which govern lives in the aggregate*' (Dickens, 1995:103).

Confronted with scientific evidence about the risk of developing a serious disease at some future date, many will see themselves as being in a position similar to the one Louisa's and thus forced to answer the question: what is the relationship between this general, statistical knowledge and *my* life? What 19th-century Louisa did not yet know, and her father was unable to express, we have learned over the past decades: the connection between "*the laws which govern lives in the aggregate*" and our personal life is established by a new perspective on life, the perspective of life management.

In industrial countries in the late 20th century, disease is no longer considered as a matter of fate, but increasingly as a risk. When fate intervenes, we may seek compensation for the victims. Social security laws have been introduced in the past to provide this, based on social insurance organised on the level of society as a whole. Risk, in the modern sense, however, is associated with action and individual responsibility (Beck, 1992; Lupton, 1999). To a large extent, we have learned to hold ourselves responsible for our health. Health promotion campaigns have no doubt contributed to this, but their efforts can hardly explain the unquestioned acceptance of this view. It seems safe to assume that there is more involved, namely a change in *ethos* with a broader background – a change in the way in which we have come to perceive ourselves, our actions and relationships.

French sociologists Luc Boltanski and Ève Chiapello have argued that a new '*ethos*' has taken hold in Western societies (Boltanski and Chiapello, 1991). It differs from the rationalist Calvinist *ethos* Max Weber had identified in his classical studies as the root of the capitalist economy and modernity (Weber, 1969). For his enquiry, Weber studied sermons of Protestant ministers from the 17th century. Boltanski and Chiapello studied management textbooks of the past decades, *i.e.* the preaches of the post-modern age.

In modern textbooks, managers are no longer depicted as the leaders of big corporations and as rationalists who rigorously follow bureaucratic rules, but as the motivators of teams of workers who concentrate on projects. The true contemporary manager is presented as the person who inspires his personnel, bypassing bureaucratic rules, and as the initiator of new projects, Boltanski and Chiapello observe. In order to fulfill this role, the manager has to continuously extend his network of contacts. In today's business-world, inspiration, innovation and an extended social network have become values in themselves.

The vocabulary and values that Boltanski and Chiapello have found in management textbooks is not confined to the world of business schools. They have spilt over into health care and the way we perceive our daily lives. For example, they are also prominently present in brochures and on the websites of patient groups. There too, we find calls to 'manage' one's disease as a 'project', and the advice to seek new contacts and to get involved with patient groups that provide mutual trust and the openness to discuss one's problems. At the same time, patients are encouraged not to let their disease or their health risk completely control their lives, but to start new 'projects' and to consciously extend their network of personal contacts. A life at risk may offer much more than fear for the future. Websites established by patient groups often tell the personal stories of people who report how their lives got new meanings after their diagnosis and how they have succeeded in enriching their relationships with friends and relatives.

Boltanski and Chiapello's bold thesis may help to understand the ease and the speed with which the management perspective on life has gained acceptance and the idea that we are responsible for our health has become common. This is a perspective that has become dominant also in other important segments of daily life, in particular in contemporary labour relations – a view, moreover, that is communicated in soap operas and popular talk shows. This is the *ethos* of the risk society.

Modern culture, the risk society, provides the rich soil in which predictive Medicine, genetic screening and future genetic diagnostics may flourish. The context needed for the new technologies to take root is already present. It would, however, be a mistake to accept uncritically the perspective on health and disease that is suggested by this context. How much influence do people really have on their future health? How much responsibility can they reasonably take for it? With all due respect to contemporary health advice and with the important exception of genetic counselling for people with a known family history of disease, we have to acknowledge that what – ironically – may be the best advice for health is seldom heard: those who want to have a long and relatively disease-free life had better be sure that they are born as the daughter of rich parents. For, even in industrial societies, socio-economic variables still explain the majority of variance in morbidity and mortality.

Twentieth-century laws that regulate the sick role and provide compensation for those who fall ill have not changed the fact that there are important differences in mortality and morbidity between the social classes. But they have provided an important buffer for those who have had the bad luck to succumb to illness: they have protected the sick from social disaster. No similar buffer exists for people at risk. There is nothing in place for those at risk that is even the approximate equivalent of the rights, care and collective services that health laws provide for the sick.

In his classic study of the sociology of religion, Max Weber observed that "interests (material and ideal), not ideas, determine human action. However: 'pictures of the world', which have been shaped by 'ideas', have often functioned like pointsmen to determine the tracks along which the dynamics of interests of action have taken their course" (Weber, 1968). Predictive medicine has brought health care onto new tracks. Gradually, we have become accustomed to a new perspective on health and disease, and have internalised a new picture of the world. No doubt this train will continue on its way for the foreseeable future. To accept that as a fact does not imply an unthinking acceptance of technological or social determinism. Although there may not be a road back, we should be on the lookout for new switches to come.

Predictive medicine and genetics present a challenge to society. Current discussions about genetics tend to focus on the technologies that will become available for diagnosis and treatment and the impact they will have. Unfortunately, the social context in which these technologies will take root has largely been taken for granted. A myopic view of technological development limits our perspective. Rather than limiting the powers of genetic technologies, the political challenge of genetics rests in critical analysis of the *ethos*, the vocabulary and values with which we approach 21st-century medicine.

Acknowledgments

Research for this article has been supported by a grant from the '*Sociale cohesie programma*' of the Netherlands Organisation for Scientific Research, NWO. I wish to thank Dr. Annemiek Nelis, Universiteit van Amsterdam, for her comments on an earlier draft of this paper.

References

Alzheimer, A., *Über Eine Eigenartige Erkrankung Der Hirnrinde, The Early Story of Alzheimer's Disease*, ed. K Bick *et al.*, New York, Rave Press, 1987 (Orig. 1907).

Beck, U., *Risk Society – Towards a New Modernity*, Trans. M. Ritter. London, SAGE Publications, 1992.

Boltanski, L. and Chiapello. E., *Le Nouvel Esprit du Capitalisme*, Paris, Gallimard-NRF Essais, 1999.

Dickens, C., *Hard Times*, London, Penguin Books, 1995 (orig. 1854).

EGE (European Group on Ethics in Science and New Technologies to the European Commission), *Genetic Testing in the Workplace*, Luxembourg, Office for Official Publications of the European Communities, 2000.

Foucault, M., *The Birth of the Clinic*, New York, Vintage Books, 1975.

Habermas, J., *Die Zukunft Der Menschlichen Natur. Auf Dem Weg Zu Einer Liberalen Eugenetik?*, Frankfurt am Main, Suhrkamp Verlag, 2001.

Horstman, K., *Public Bodies, Private Lives – the Historical Construction of Life Insurance, Health Risks, and Citizenship in the Netherlands, 1880 – 1920*, Rotterdam, Erasmus Publishing, 2001.

HGAC (Human Genetics Advisory Commission), *The Implications of Genetic Testing for Employment*, 1999, available at: http://www.doh.gov.uk/hgac/.

Kitcher, P., *The Lives to Come – the Genetic Revolution and Human Possibilities*, London, Penguin Books, 1996.

Lupton, D., *Risk*, London, Routledge, 1999.

Morison-Bogorod, M. *et al.*, "Alzheimer Disease Comes of Age," *Journal of the American Medical Association*, 277.10 March 12, 1997:837 ff.

OECD, *Genetic Testing – Policy Issues for the New Millennium*, Paris, OECD, 2000.

Porter, D. and Porter, R., *Patient's Progress – Doctors and Doctoring in Eighteenth-Century England*, Oxford, Polity Press, 1989.

Schulte, P.A. and DeBord, D.G., "Public Health Assessment of Genetic Information in the Occupational Setting," in Muin J. Khoury, Wylie Burke and Elizabeth Thomson (eds.), *Genetics and Public Health in the 21st Century:*

Using Genetic Information to Improve Health and Prevent Disease, New York, Oxford University Press, 2000.

Temple, Larissa K. F., *et al.*, "Defining Disease in the Genomics Era," Science 293.5531 (2001):807-808.

Van Damme, K., and Casteleyn, L., "Genetic Susceptibility and Health at Work," 2002, available at: http://www.genetic-testing-and-work.be.

Weber, M., *Die Protestantische Ethik Und Der Geist Des Kapitalismus*, München und Hamburg, Siebenstern Taschenbuch Verlag, 1969 (orig. 1905).

Weber, M., *Gesammelte Aufsätze Zur Wissenschaftslehre*, Tübingen, J.C.B. Mohr Paul Siebeck, 1968.

CHAPTER 2

Ethical, Legal and Practical Aspects of Genetic Testing at Work

Marja SORSA and Karel VAN DAMME

1. Introduction

Genetic technologies, along with the applications to which they are put and the benefits and risks ensuing from their development are increasingly in the forefront of public debates relating to advances in the fields of science and new technology. This is a new incentive for the scientific community to intensify communication with the general public, administrators and decision makers, all of whom wish to be involved in making decisions which might well concern their future and well-being. In an ever more competitive economic context, employers may have an increasing interest in the possibility of selecting the best, fittest and healthiest job-applicants or employees on the basis of their molecular genetic profile. The presumption is that genetic tests can predict future health outcomes and consequently, future levels of sick leave and lower work efficiency, both of which have serious conse-quences for business profitability. Is this an illusion or a real prospect in the near future?

The extraordinary speed at which molecular genetic techniques have been developed since the launching of the human genome projects less than a decade ago has been one of the most exciting features of the area of study. The precision and speed of the analyses, the tiny amounts of DNA material needed for analysis, the automation of the methods and the decreasing cost of the analyses has put an enormous speculative commercial pressure in development of "easy" genetic tests and test kits. These are intended, not only for diagnostic purposes but also for the identification of potential susceptibility to disease. Commercial genetic laboratories and the producers of tests have started a new predictive medicine industry which does not necessarily follow scientific quality criteria, medical responsibility codes or ethical principles. Neither is respect for privacy or confidentiality guaranteed. Cases of false positive and false negative test results, as well as discrimination based on potential genetic risk in health insurance, job applications and in child adoption have been documented and debated, particularly in the United States (see *e.g.* Nowak, 1994; European Group on Ethics, 2003). Furthermore, the ethics of equal access to high quality genetic testing services has been questioned, especially by genetics expert groups in the European Union (Kristoffersson *et al.*, 1999).

Within the occupational health activities, whether research-oriented or as part of occupational medicine practices, the term 'genetic testing' is usually understood to include all analyses on bio-samples from workers (typically blood, urine, skin, other tissue or cell samples) designed to identify alterations in the genetic material – inherited or induced – in the person to be tested. In the latter case, genetic testing is used to identify evidence of induced changes, *e.g.* due to work-related exposure to genotoxic agents (see review of methods and applications in Sorsa 1996). In cases of repeated analyses, we speak rather of *genetic monitoring*. In some cases genetic monitoring may be regarded as part of occupational health surveillance, *e.g.* chromosomal aberration analyses or micronucleus test for those working with ionising radiation. Positive findings in genetic monitoring should lead to occupational safety precautions and prevention of the causative work-related exposure.

Molecular genetic techniques allow genetic testing to be performed in order to identify specific inherited conditions, diseases or susceptibilities to disorders in bio-samples from which the person's DNA (or specific gene product) can be extracted. These genetic testing activities on otherwise healthy persons may be called *genetic screening* and they are thought to be predictive for inherited conditions that may or may not relate to an occupational disease. Genetic screening tests may be performed either as part of an employees' occupational health program or as pre-employment testing of job-applicants. Both the objectives and the ethical issues involved are different for genetic monitoring and genetic screening when undertaken as part of occupational safety and health practices (see Table 1).

Table 1. Main differences in the application of genetic monitoring and genetic screening in occupational health practices

GENETIC MONITORING	GENETIC SCREENING
Timing Performed during employment	*Timing* Performed pre-employment or during employment
Tools Identification of exposure-related effects	*Tools* Identification of susceptibility to an occupational disease exposure or to any other disease at a later date
Aims Identification of hazard at work	*Aims* Exclusion of employees or job-applicants at increased risk of disease later in life
Input in risk assessment	Job replacement for susceptible workers.
Decrease of exposure levels. Replacement of hazardous compounds in the workplace. Lowering of limit values.	Individual genetic counselling

As is evident from Table 1, the ethical challenge relates especially to genetic screening and predictive testing of healthy individuals.

2. Application of Genetic Testing in Employment

Employers' main interest in the use of modern genetic screening tools is most likely to be in seeking to lower health-related costs in their enterprises. This is especially so in societies with a private health insurance system. The reasoning of the employers who use genetic tests in pre-employment screening and 'weeding' may be that predictive information from genetic analyses ensures healthier employees with lower sickness rates who are liable to retire later. However, the scientific basis of predictability of present tests is thin, as most diseases are, in fact, multifactorial and are caused by complex interactions among genes and between the genes and environmental factors. For these and other reasons, the whole enterprise may well be misconceived (see Casteleyn *et al.*, 1997).

The number of genetic screening tests available is actually still quite limited. The tests so far available have limited sensitivity and specificity so that a number of false negatives and false positives lead to misclassifications. Even in tests for monogenetic hereditary diseases that are well-characterised, performed by both public and private genetic laboratories, unexpected errors do occur. This has emerged as a feature of testing in quality assurance studies, both in European and US laboratories (see surveys coordinated by the OECD, *e.g.* "Genetic Testing. Policy Issues for the New Millennium," 2000). The relevance of genetic tests with respect to disease outcome for any multifactorial disease is also highly questionable. Although the prices of test kits are expected to fall, the tests are still quite costly, partly due to monopoly system under which the patents are licensed.

At present, the concern and debate aroused by genetic screening of employees or of job applicants, is quite clearly out of proportion with the reality of the paucity/meagre levels of genetic testing actually being performed by enterprises and occupational health services. Large-scale surveys performed in the US by the Office of Technology Assessment in 1982 and 1989 revealed some use of genetic testing (mainly cytogenetic surveillance) in large companies (1.6 and 5.0% of respondents in respective years) and a clear potential interest in future years (Froneberg, 2003). However, in the survey conducted in 2001 by the American Management Association, a clear decline in performing any kind of medical testing was seen and genetic testing was reported only in 2 out of some 1600 companies (Froneberg, 2003).

In Europe, there has been no extensive surveying on the subject of the use of work-related genetic testing. Although genetic monitoring (cytogenetic surveillance for structural chromosome aberrations or related types of effect) has been used in some countries – among nuclear power plant workers for as a biological dosimeter, for example – and a great number of studies have been undertaken on members of various occupations for research purposes, genetic screening as a routine practice is known only in the UK. The Royal Air Force has long screened for the sickle cell trait, on the assumption that hemolytic crisis in sickle cell carriers flying in low oxygen pressure conditions constituted a particular danger. According to the report of the European Group on Ethics report (EGE, 2003) the UK Ministry of Defence has discontinued the practice. The EGE further reports the results of a survey carried out by the Institute of Directors in the UK in 2000, in which only 2 out of 353 directors reported that their enterprises use genetic tests routinely, while 4 apply them in special cases only.

One could distinguish two different purposes for performing genetic screening of employees: (1) the prediction of future health (without any specific connection to the work environment) or (2) as an indicator of specific genetic susceptibility in relation to the hazardous exposures in the work place (see Table 1).

In the former category, the future health of the employee or the job applicant forms part of his/her private and confidential health information and may not be used for occupational health purposes unless it can be shown that the health of the worker, in view of the nature of his/her duties, is likely to endanger the safety of third parties. The decision on fitness for work can be fraught with difficulties which arise from the need to respect both the patient's medical confidentiality and his/her right to know – or indeed, not to know – about the probability of future health problems. As mentioned earlier, the results of a single genetic screening test may lack accuracy, even for the monogenetic disease conditions (*e.g.* sickle cell anemia, Huntington's disease or cystic fibrosis). The usefulness of tests which seek to predict the appearance of diseases caused by polygenic and complex environmental factors is limited (*e.g.* type I diabetes, hereditary breast cancer, heart disease). The association is further weakened by uncertainties in the manifestation of the disease, its severity, progression and timing.

As regards the second purpose for screening mentioned above, rapid developments in the DNA microarray techniques now allow the simultaneous screening for several hundred of genetic traits so that the "genetic profile" of an employee may be reviewed for special susceptibilities in relation to workplace hazards, *e.g.* genotoxic chemicals or physical agents. Some evidence about the role of genetic predisposition factors has been reported *e.g.* UV and ionising radiation associated cancers (some repair deficiency genes), aromatic amines and bladder cancer (N-acetyltransferase gene deficiency), beryllium and pulmonary allergic hypertension (specific HLA variant gene), organic dust and chronic obstructive pulmonary disease (alpha-1-antitrypsine gene deficiency). However, the general conclusion tends to be that, particularly in the case of metabolic susceptibility genes in prediction of cancer risk, individual predictions are possible only very rarely, and even then, only for those who have mutated high-penetrance cancer susceptibility genes and who are members of cancer-prone families (see *e.g.* Shields and Harris, 2000).

3. Genetic Impairment for Work?

The removal of hazardous agents from the workplace and the prevention of worker exposures is very clearly the primary solution taken by the employers and the occupational safety and health system at present. In very rare special cases which include the obvious increased health hazard to third parties or a scientifically proven association of a specific genetic constitution with unpreventable risk of exposure to a work-related causative agent it, could be found ethically acceptable to use genetic data to prevent an employee or others being exposed to a known health risk. Colour blindness in train drivers and airplane pilots is one of the few documented examples of exclusion at the job application stage due to a genetic impairment (tested by a phenotypic vision test). Job applicants may have been excluded from other occupations but these cases are not well documented, nor do they really bear the scientific causality proof showing the connection between the genetic impairment increasing the risk to health at work. Some recent cases from the US are often cited: the Lawrence Berkeley Laboratory testing for the sickle cell trait and the Burlington Northern Santa Fe Railroad Company testing for chromosome damage (cited *e.g.* in the EGE report, 2003). In both cases, the companies were sued for discrimination and these claims were settled out of court, with compensation being paid to the claimants.

Even if the knowledge of large public health diseases, such as type II diabetes, arteriosclerosis, mental disorders, arthritis, allergies and many cancers is rapidly increasing, their genetic basis is still poorly understood and the etiology is complex, including gene interactions, as well as the influences of lifestyle, diet and environmental factors. Thus, based both on the principles of scientific uncertainty and on the irrelevance of the potential illness to the person's job or work place hazards, routine occupational testing practices unrelated to occupational health risks should not be allowed.

In cases where no legal restrictions apply (see section 8 on legal development), several criteria have to be fulfilled and carefully considered before planning the use of genetic testing in work-related health hazard situations:

- Is the condition in question a serious and preventable disease?
- What is the true and relative risk of the subject developing the disease?
- Is there experimental evidence to support the association of work-related exposure with the appearance of the disease?
- Is there any epidemiologic or case report evidence about causality in occupational exposure situations?
- Is the genetic testing method valid, reliable and accurate?
- Can the hazardous agent be removed from the work place or can the subjects' exposure be reduced through avoidance measures?
- Could the disease be prevented by more effective health surveillance?
- Is there an association between the prevalence of the genetic risk factor and specific populations or groups of persons?

- How many employees might be affected by a negative test result and what are the possibilities for job replacement?
- What can be done to prevent exposure and to rearrange the distribution of tasks
- What arrangements are in place to guarantee the subjects' privacy and to maintain their confidentiality?
- Is the employee's consent given on the basis of a full understanding of the issues involved? Has the consent been given freely and without pressure or coercion on the part of the employer?
- Do negative consequences attach to an employee's refusal to give consent?

The reason for answering these questions is to ensure that where genetic testing is undertaken, its primary purpose is to protect the health and safety of employees and thus to prevent – rather than predict the appearance of disease.

4. Ethical Principles

The general ethical principles involved in the analysis of work-related genetic testing have been touched on above and are discussed in detail by other authors in this publication. Although the 'Georgetown ethical principles for medical action' (*beneficence, non-maleficience, autonomy* and *justice*) (Beauchamps *et al.*, 1979) are respected in most human societies, their weighing and balancing may change with time and with regard to different stake-holders.

Both the International Labour Organisation (ILO) and generally the codes of good occupational health practice cite *opportunity for employment, job security, health, self-esteem and privacy* as items of basic concern in discussing genetic testing in the workplace. The ILO's Code of Practice on Protection of Workers' Personal Data (1997) specifically states that medical personal data may only be collected as needed, *i.e.* to determine whether the worker is fit for a particular employment, to fulfill the requirements of occupational health and safety, and to determine entitlements or grant social benefits. Genetic screening should be prohibited or limited to exceptional cases explicitly authorised by national legislation. The subjection of workers to genetic testing may not be left to employers' discretion. These statements are reflected in some recent national legislation on occupational testing (see section number 8 on legal development).

5. Ethical Contradictions in the Workplace

There is a basic difference in viewpoints on genetic testing between employers and employees, especially in those countries where employment is linked to the private health insurance system, like in the US (see *e.g.* Draper, 1991). In these countries, genetic monitoring is generally considered as more acceptable by the workers and labour organisations. Genetic screening is generally not acceptable to employees, mainly because of fears of discrimination, but it is frequently considered a future possibility by employers in order to reduce health care costs.

At the job application stage, the employer selects the applicant best fit to perform the tasks required. According to codes of practice (if not legislation) all medical examinations, including pre-employment examinations, are limited in principle to measuring the ability of the employee to perform the functions related to the job at the time of the examination. Discrimination in employment on the basis of race, colour, sex, religion, political opinion, national extraction or social origin is in many countries prohibited under the terms of the constitution, specific legislation and international convention. The spirit of this prohibition would appear to include discrimination based on genetic factors, even though genes naturally play an important role in many individual characteristics and personality.

Concerning possible genetic testing as part of occupational health services, there are several potential sources for conflicting opinions:

- differences in employees' state of health;
- trust in respect for the privacy and confidentiality of personal medical data;
- differences in interests and beliefs of the various parties and stakeholders;
- differences in dealing with uncertainty about the science base;
- uneven distribution of knowledge;
- differences in concern over preventive action.

A potential source of conflict derives from the vigorous marketing of genetic tests. In order to generate profits, commercialisation and mass marketing are essential for the producers of the tests. Consequently, the pharmaceutical industry and the private medical sector 'talk up' the future potential of the "post genomic era" producing cheap genetic test kits for everybody's use. Internet marketing is already encouraging the use of test kits. Unfortunately these are distributed without reliable information or any medical or genetic counselling and their accuracy, validity and ethical acceptability are highly questionable.

It is quite obvious that long-term planning, open discussion and informative debate between the parties are necessary before embarking – if at all – on genetic testing in the workplace.

6. Dilemma of Informed Consent

The principle of consent is part of the principle of individual autonomy which has long been applied in biomedical research concerning human subjects, as well as in clinical practice. However, the freedom of the consenting subject is sometimes questionable. It is especially problematic with persons not able to give a free and informed consent (minors, elderly persons with dementia, unconscious patients, seriously ill patients, patients before operations or medical treatment *etc.*). Equally, prisoners, soldiers or those who form part of a strongly hierarchical system may act under pressure so that the consent given is not actually free. The same may be true also for job applicants or employees in insecure employment contracts. While free consent is sometimes not guaranteed in research settings, it would be a matter of serious concern if it were to be used as a regulatory principle in occupational health practices. This issue is discussed briefly in the next section.

In research settings, the consent of the subject should be informed by written and oral information explaining the reasons for, and potential consequences of, genetic testing. This information should be made available before the start of tests. It is essential that the possibility to withdraw from participation, as well as the right not to know the results is made clear to the subjects. The uncertainty factors in the interpretation of the results should be explained, especially concerning genetic testing used at the research stage. There should also be a possibility for genetic counselling, as well as occupational health and safety counselling, after the study is completed.

The information given should include the main stakeholders and be given in an understandable way to all. The usual stakeholders in the occupational setting are: the workers, occupational health units, employers and the scientific community. The most common questions to be answered are the following:

- What is being studied?
- Why the study is being performed?
- What are the risks involved?
- How is confidentiality to be ensured?
- What are the methods to be used?

- What are the plans for prevention of hazardous exposure?
- What is the scientific relevance of the study?

When consent is given, it should be in writing and preferably well in advance of the actual testing. By this time, the employee should be able to answer affirmatively to the following questions:

- Has the information given been understood?
- Has the information given been comprehensive and trustworthy?
- Has the decision to give consent been independent?

Confidentiality and privacy are the key elements in any physician-patient relationship, and this is also true in research settings. Genetic screening differs from other medical testing primarily in that the result may concern not only the subject her/himself, but also her/his parents, children and future generations and other family members. This has a special significance in screening for hereditary diseases, but naturally, also other genes are inherited under similar the same laws of heredity.

7. Scenarios in Occupational Health Practices

According to the concrete items of concern, based on ethical principles, protecting both health and the employment of every single worker or job candidate should be the guiding paradigm for all actions by occupational health services. This includes that priority should be given to improving working conditions, rather than excluding a worker from (access to) job.

Several questions must be answered in order to assess the compliance of practices with the ethical principles:

- Who makes the decision?
- Upon what issue is the decision made?
- Whom does the decision concern?
- Why is the decision made?
- How is the decision made?
- On what ground is the decision made?
- What consequences may the decision have?

One could clarify the issue by distinguishing two extremes. The first of these gives full power to the employer in a society with social security almost exclusively dependent upon current employment. In the second, the legislature decides on the acceptability of practices following consultation with the social partners involved and the societal context is marked by a well-developed social security system which is independent of employment.

In the first case, the employer has full power to decide upon the fitness of the worker for the job as it is. Selection of the fittest with the aim of reducing absenteeism and private insurance costs are major goals of the employer's policy. An occupational health physician or nurse does the testing on behalf of the employer and in the way the employer requires it to be done. His choice is based on the expected benefits for the company or on the criteria of the private insurance company for calculating the premium based on the expected risk. The consequences of such a policy would lead to systematic exclusion of many employees who are assumed to be more vulnerable or do not comply with particular fitness standards. Due to the lack of social security provisions independent of current employment, exclusion may easily lead to poverty of the employee and those who depend on his/her income.

In the second scenario, the legislator – following consultation with the social partners – decides not only on the criteria for fitness for the worker concerned, but also on the duties of the employer, on the criteria for considering a worker or job candidate as unfit. In fact, legislation decides on the whole system: how priority is given to the protection of both health and the right to access to work of every individual worker. The legal system decides who can do medical testing and the role of the occupational health professionals. The legislator also decides to what extent and under which circumstances the occupational health physician will act in an advisory or decision-making capacity and cannot be overruled by the employer. Scientific relevance to the protection of the employee's health is the guiding principle for testing. Adapting the job or working conditions to the capacities of the employee and avoiding that a person's exposure to working conditions which he cannot handle, are the goals. Where exclusion from job is the only solution, social security systems prevent that this would lead to poverty.

Informed consent by the employee concerned is often put forward as a "magic trick" to make any system acceptable (see Section 6). Both extreme scenarios give us a better view on the possible consequences of applying the principle of informed consent in occupational health practices. In the first scenario, adding informed consent does not in any way affect the ultimate full decisional autonomy of the employer, who decides whatever he wants. Logically, the employer may easily consider refusal of a test for whatever reason as synonymous with exclusion. In this context of power inequality, informed consent is an irrelevant solution. In the second scenario, adding informed consent, and thus a refusal of the employee or job candidate to be tested, does not allow the occupational health physician to recommend employment under conditions as such a recommendation may cause health damage to relatively more vulnerable persons.

There are different systems in between these extremes. It is unclear how a system that deviates significantly from the second scenario would allow one to respect the principle of protecting both health and employment.

Within the European Union, occupational health is facing a new challenge (Van Damme *et al.*, 2003). Occupational health policies have evolved during the last century from survival of the fittest to a system of social protection, which in some Member States was very close to the second scenario mentioned in the previous paragraph. Well-developed systems of medical surveillance, including systematic biological monitoring for workers at risk, are accessible to most employees in several Member States. The basic principle consists of striving to adapt the working conditions to the abilities of the workers, with the aim of protecting both the health and employment of every worker.

In recent years, the EU single market strategy has been the driving force for waves of necessary standardisation procedures. This entails the idea of a standardised occupational health policy. The unfortunate threat is that no incentive will be left for the employer to adapt working conditions to the abilities of the individual workers. Instead, the paradigm is a flexible workforce with workers who are selected for their compatibility with what could be called the standardised working conditions. Employers' liability would be limited to compliance with a set of workplace standards, which will refer to a (non-existent) 'standard worker'. New medical technologies, such as genetic tests, are believed to allow for the selection of the fittest worker, through prediction of individual risk. Goals of a standardisation policy include not only the reduction of occupational diseases, but also the reduction of absenteeism and/or insurance costs. Such a policy would inevitably lead to the exclusion of more workers and is also likely to be based on scientifically irrational grounds. Based on the above discussion, it remains to be seen what place will be given in the EU to genetic testing in relation to the two development scenarios.

If this evolution is not anticipated, selection of the fittest, not social protection, will be the goal. This resembles very much the policy of survival of the fittest in the early industrialised world. In contrast with this tendency, both the ILO principles and the ICOH International Code for Occupational Health Professionals call for social protection of every individual worker.

8. Legal Developments in Regulating Genetic Testing at Work

A fundamental principle of European legal structure, which also informs occupational safety and health practices, is the respect of confidentiality. This is vital in guaranteeing confidentiality of all medical data, including genetic data.

In many European countries there is no specific legislation on the use of genetic testing at work, but it is covered by legislation regarding privacy, confidentiality and patient's rights in medical examinations and research (see Table 2). A wide general consensus seems to exist that employers should not be able to use results of genetic tests to exclude individuals from employment or advancement of their career on the basis of genetic predisposition to future disease (CDBI, Council of Europe, 2001).

The European Group on Ethics (EGE) in its Opinion No.18 (2003) has taken a stand to recommend increasing harmonisation of legislation within the European Union, especially considering the goal of free movement of labour within the EU and the fact that the "lack of adequate protection may hurt trust, mutual respect and professionalism in the relationship between employers and employees" and consequently, European business as a whole.

Several countries, following the articles in the Council of Europe Convention on Human Rights and Biomedicine (1997), have adopted legislation permitting genetic testing only where it has a medical aim or serves a medical research purpose (*e.g.* Sweden, Spain, Georgia) and placing restrictions on the collection and processing of genetic data in the workplace (*e.g.* Netherlands, Luxembourg, Greece).

Although different traditions exist in regard to rights and regulations between workers and employers in different parts of the world, they should not stand in the way of the simultaneous enforcement of basic ethical principles and the development of legislation to protect the right of access to work, the right to health and the right to privacy.

Table 2. Legislative action on genetic testing and employment at national level in some European countries

Country	Name of Law	Year passed	Main restrictive element
Austria	Gene Technology Act	1995, 1998	Prohibits employers to collect or demand genetic test data
Belgium	Law on medical examinations related to employment	2003	Prohibits genetic testing except if imposed by Royal Decree in very specific circumstances, and prohibits any testing done by other persons than the legal occupational health physician
Denmark	Act on the Use of Health Information on the Labour Market	1996	Health examinations must focus on present health condition relevant to the employees' work
Estonia	Human Genes Research Act	2001	Employers are prohibited to collect genetic data or require tissue or DNA samples from employees or job applicants
Finland	Privacy at Work Act	2001	Employers are prohibited to require genetic testing or ask for information about such tests from employees
France	Act on discrimination for reasons of health or infirmity (1990)	Amendment of 2002	Prohibition based on genetic characteristics or genetic predisposition to a disease

References

Beauchamps, T.L. and Childress T.F., *Principles of Biomedical Ethics*, New York, Oxford University Press, 1979.

Casteleyn, L. and Van Damme, K., "Analysis of Practices in Occupational Health: Susceptibility testing in Pre-placement Examinations," Proceedings of the International Symposium 'Ethical and Social Principles in Occupational Health Practice', Finland, December 1997, Research reports 21, Helsinki 1998, 8-16.

Council of Europe, Convention on Human Rights and Biomedicine, *Directorate of Legal Affairs*, DIR/JUR, 1996, 14, Strasbourg, November, 1996.

Council of Europe, Steering Committee on Bioethics, *Working Party on Human Genetics*, CDBI-CO-GT4, 2001, 9.

Draper, E., *Risky Business. Genetic Testing and Exclusionary Practices in the Hazardous Workplace*, New York, Cambridge University Press, 1991, 1-315.

EGE. (European Group on Ethics in Science and New Technologies to the European Commission), *Opinion on the Ethical Aspects of Genetic Testing in the Workplace*, Opinion No.18, 28 July 2003, European Communities, Luxembourg.

Froneberg, B., "Ethical Aspects of Genetic Testing at the Workplace. Position and activities of the International Labour Organisation," Presentation at the EGE meeting 15 April 2003 and cited in the EGE Opinion Report 18, 2003.

Gottlieb, S., "US Employer Agrees to Stop Genetic Testing," *British Medical Journal 322*, 2001, 449-450.

ILO (International Labour Organisation), *Protection of Workers' Personal Data. An ILO Code of Practice*, Geneva, Switzerland, 1997.

ILO (International Labour Organisation), "Technical and Ethical Guidelines for Workers' Health Surveillance," *Occupational Health Series* 72, Geneva, Switzerland, 1998.

Kristofferson, U., Rosén K.-E. and Sorup, P., "Promoting Equal Accessibility of Genetic Testing Services of High Quality in the EU through the Development of European Standards," The (Institute of Prospective Technological Studies) *IPTS Report* 35, 1999, 20-24.

Nowak, R., "Genetic Testing Set for Takeoff," *Science* 265, 1994, 464-467.

OECD (Organisation for Economic Co-operation and Development), "Genetic Testing. Policy Issues for the New Millennium," *Science and Innovation*, Paris, France, 2000, 1-76.

Shields, P.G. and Harris, C.C., "Cancer Risk and Low-penetrance Susceptibility Genes in Gene-Environment Interactions," *Journal of Clinical Oncology* 18, 2000, 2309-2315.

Sorsa, M., "Genetic Monitoring: Experiences, Possibilities and Applications in Occupational Health Practices," *International Journal of Occupational and Environmental Health* 2, 1996, 554-556.

Van Damme, K. and Casteleyn, L., "Current Scientific, Ethical and Social Issues of Biomonitoring in the European Union," *Toxicology Letters* 144, 2003, 117-126.

PART II

INFORMATION TECHNOLOGY AND PRIVACY AT WORK

CHAPTER 3

New Monitoring
and Surveillance Technology

Simon ROGERSON and Mary PRIOR

1. Introduction

People are of prime importance to every organisation and the way in which they are treated can make the difference between the success or failure of a venture. Employees have always been subjected to checking and monitoring. However, Information and Communication Technologies (ICT) are now prevalent in most workplaces and are used in an attempt to increase efficiency and effectiveness in a vast range of business processes. The power and flexibility of these technologies have presented new ways of auditing employees' work. For not only has electronic monitoring replaced cumbersome tools such as timesheets and clocking in cards; it offers the possibility of monitoring a much greater variety of performance and resource usage parameters in detail and in a continuous fashion. It has been argued that the use of electronic forms of monitoring and surveillance is not simply 'more of the same' but qualitatively different from the use of more traditional means. Sewell and Barker (2001) point out that ICT not only increase the reach or immediacy of familiar forms of surveillance but also, "enable new forms to operate that we have less experience of containing." This presents a potential tension between the employer's desire to ensure their employees are working effectively and the employees' human rights.

It is worth at this point discussing what is meant by the terms, 'monitoring' and 'surveillance'. Botan and McCreadie (1993) note the distinction made by Attewell (1987) and conclude that the term 'monitoring' is generic and can be applied to all automated collecting of information about work, regardless of purpose. Monitoring produces information that can be used for everything from setting bonuses and keeping track of inventory to controlling individual employees. On the other hand, the term 'surveillance' more narrowly refers to a relationship between some authority and those whose behaviour it wishes to control (Rule and Brantley, 1992). Monitoring generates the information used in surveillance. All surveillance incorporates monitoring, but not all monitoring is used for surveillance. Lankshear and Mason (2001) use the term, 'surveillance-capable technologies' which usefully captures a key feature; questions concerning their use may only arise after they are in place. Often systems installed for one ostensible purpose, such as the protection of property from theft in a retail outlet, are found to be equally useful for a completely different purpose such as the observation of staff behaviour towards customers. Indeed function creep has always been a prevalent trait of ICT. Such creep often occurs without due consideration and proper evaluation.

Thus new technologies make it possible for employers to monitor many aspects of their employees' work, particularly where this involves the use of telephones, electronic and voice mail, computer terminals and the internet. Accepting regulation of the workplace exists, there are however still instances, unless organisational policy specifically states otherwise (and even then this is not assured), where an employer may listen, watch and read their employees' workplace communications.

2. Context of Electronic Monitoring

There are a variety of forms of electronic monitoring in place and a variety of reasons for their use. The scope of their use may vary, as does the employee population subject to monitoring. The relationship between these factors and their consequence for the relationship between employee and employer is illustrated in Figure 1.

Figure 1. Five Elements of Workplace Monitoring

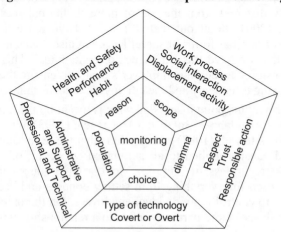

Reasons may include the need to conform to health and safety requirements in certain industries which, it can be argued, are both legitimate and beneficial to all stakeholders. Where the reason is for monitoring employee performance or habits, the legitimacy of this practice may be questioned. Which aspects of performance are being monitored, by whom, and for what purposes? Who has access to and control over the information gathered about individuals? Are the individuals aware of the monitoring?

With respect to the employee populations, one characteristic of electronic surveillance is that it opens up to scrutiny the work of groups of employees who may not previously have been subject to close levels of monitoring. The traditional factory or office floor enabled manual or clerical workers used to be subject to closer scrutiny than their supervisors or other types of professional or managerial staff. Now anybody whose work involves the use of telecommunication and computer equipment, no matter where they are located, or who works in an environment where access is controlled by smart Cards or Closed Circuit Television (CCTV) can find not only their work output but also their activities while at work being monitored. Ironically, at the same time as there has been decentralisation and devolution of responsibility for tactical decision-making in many organisations, there has been an increase in the level of centralised strategic control and surveillance in order to ensure that the whole workforce remains focussed on the organisation's goals (Sewell and Wilkinson, 1992). Clement (1992) claims, 'as long as organisations face an increasingly competitive, turbulent environment while work grows ever more complex, abstract, spatially distributed, and computerised, the pressure on managers to take advantage of these new panoptic capabilities for control can only intensify'.

Electronic monitoring technologies can measure only certain aspects of an employee's work, such as the length and number of calls taken, the time spent at a terminal, the number of keystrokes, their movements about a building. These parameters encompass only a limited part of the entire scope of an employee's work. The contributions to a productive working environment of key elements of the work process such as social interaction are in danger of being under-estimated or completely ignored. Monitoring may detect an employee apparently engaged in more 'displacement' activity than others or greater than some prescribed level. This could lead to the assumption by a manager or supervisor that such an employee is less productive.

The choice as to whether workplace monitoring and surveillance should be covert or overt tends to be driven by the preceding factors of the reason for it, its scope and the population. Monitoring for the legitimate purpose of meeting health and safety requirements, for example, would be most effective if the employee populations are fully aware of its purpose and scope. Efforts to survey employees' social interactions may be more likely to be attempted covertly.

Decisions taken about the reasons for, extent of, approach to and subjects of monitoring and surveillance may have profound consequences on the relationship between the employer and employee. Indeed they may undermine the basic principles and values of respect, trust and responsible action.

3. Examples of Typical Monitoring

It is useful at this point to consider some typical proprietary products and the use made of such products. In doing this it is recognised that there are also some systems which provide monitoring functions discovered through implementation and are based upon their reuse of system capabilities. The monitoring capabilities of cookies and mobile phones are typical examples.

The choice of technology for workplace monitoring is vast. The manner in which such technology is marketed varies considerably. For example software acquisition choices can be split into three broad categories. The product approach is where monitoring software is offered as a product devoid of any ancillary services. The service approach is where monitoring software is offered as an element of a comprehensive package to address all aspects of surveillance and monitoring strategy. The embedded approach is where monitoring and surveillance facilities are included as additional functions in an application package and marketed as added product value. Examples of these approaches are now briefly described.

Product Approach

At the time of writing Spector Pro[1] was one of the market leaders in monitoring and surveillance software for PCs. It is indicative of this type of software both in the way it is marketed and its functionality. Marketing strategy promotes a culture of mistrust with slogans such as "When you absolutely need to know everything they are doing online" and "Even when they delete their e-mail, Spector Pro will keep a secret copy for you to review." This is supported by the functionality of the

---

[1] See www.spectorsoft.com.

software that enables many aspects of online work to be monitored. These include e-mail recording, chat and instant message recording, keystroke recording, website recording, visual snapshot recording and keyword detection. The software allows groups or individuals to be targeted. This monitoring can be set up in stealth mode which the vendor describes as monitoring that "is completely hidden from everyone except those with authorised access. It will not appear in the Windows System Tray, Desktop, Task Manager or Add/Remove Programs Menu." This type of approach seems commonplace. For example, another leading product e-Surveillor[2] provides a comprehensive range of monitoring facilities which includes logging all text typed, programs operated and files modified that is invisible and undetectable from those being monitored. It is marketed with slogans such as, "now you can see everything that they do," "secretly record everything that is typed" and "get the proof you need."

Service Approach

One of the market leaders for corporate online monitoring strategies is SurfControl.[3] The company offers a wide range of interrelated Internet filtering and monitoring products that link with an up to date database of blocked websites. Unlike Spector Pro and e-Surveillor, SurfControl offers a comprehensive business proposition by combining surveillance and monitoring software with an online knowledge base (SurfControl Resource Center) and strategy support service. SurfControl argue that, "Internet connectivity at the office also creates desktop temptations that, for many employees, are too hard to resist." Therefore businesses must mitigate the risk of productivity loss, bandwidth loss and legal liability by having effective monitoring software to back up an acceptable use policy. SurfControl point out that whilst users' privacy must be protected there has to be a balance with "the assertion that corporate e-mail boxes and IT infrastructure are corporate assets." They advocate a strategy that begins with developing an acceptable use policy, then a user education programme before finally implementing automatic filtering, surveillance and monitoring.

---

[2] See www.e-surveiller.com.

[3] See www.surfcontrol.com.

Embedded Approach

With the desire of organisations to "track" employees many software applications provide extra functionality to satisfy such requirements. For example, Heuthes[4] is a major software supplier for private companies, banks and financial institutions in Poland. One product that it offers is ISOF, which is an Internet-based corporate service system. It provides geographically dispersed companies with a simple way of developing an integrated IT system. Heuthes explains that, "It is excellent for enterprises with widespread organisation structure, owning numerous branches, affiliates and warehouses in several locations and employing many mobile workers (*e.g.* Sale Representatives)." The ISOF product description states that, "ISOF, which helps planning and controlling, is especially liked by the bosses and firm management. It makes possible the observation of all events happening within the firm. Even being far away from the office, one can check the sales, stock level and see who is currently at work." When used with sales representatives the systems log three states: work, break and travel. Each person is responsible for logging any change in state. A report is produced for each person giving a detailed time analysis. Heuthes explained that time data can be changed by the system administrator to overcome any data inaccuracies and that the system administrator, as well as line managers, had access to the time analysis report. Heuthes staff appeared to have no interest or understanding of the employment and privacy rights related to this type of embedded surveillance and monitoring function.

Applications of products such as Spector Pro, e-Surveillor, SurfControl and ISOF seem to be driven by a combination of usage management, legal compliance and culture forming. This is illustrated by the following two case studies. There appears to be a tendency to consider employees as costly liabilities susceptible to the draw of the Internet rather than a trustworthy resource.

Case 1 – Servisair

Servisair UK Ltd is a part of the largest independent airport ground handling company in the world.[5] It has 12,000 employees in 109 locations within 14 countries. The company annually handles half a million tonnes of cargo and 55 million passengers on 600,000 flights. The company is heavily reliant upon Internet and e-mail resources and consequently undertook a risk assessment of these facilities. It was

---

[4]   See www.heuthes.pl.

[5]   See www.surfcontrol.com/general/assets/case_studies/Servisair_0203.pdf.

reported that, "Hugh Foster, Servisair's Systems Support Analyst real-ised that for the company to get the most from its online access it needed to take the appropriate steps to protect employees and the company from the potential problems posed by unmanaged Internet and e-mail use in the workplace." This paternalistic stance of protecting employees is surprising given "Servisair had only experienced isolated incidents in the past." The company, "wanted to take a proactive stance and use a sophisticated technology solution to ensure that the company did all that it could to promote a responsible Web and e-mail culture."

Case 2 – The Property Advisers to the Civil Estate (PACE)

The Property Advisers to the Civil Estate (PACE) is a Government agency of the Office of Government Commerce (OGC) in the UK, specializing in property management owned or used by the Government. […] Internet fa-cilities were provided to allow PACE staff to access and retrieve informa-tion relevant to their work and as a means of communicating both within government and in the private sector.

The management within PACE were concerned that this access may be abused but there appeared to be no evidence to support this concern. This potential abuse was used as the justification to install surveillance and monitoring software. PACE believe that, "the mere fact that em-ployees are aware that they are being monitored has acted as a deterrent to abuse of the system [and] that PACE is saving a significant amount of money on time that would previously have been productivity loss." No evidence has been put forward to substantiate this claim.[6]

These examples serve as warning. Monitoring and surveillance must not simply occur because there are enabling products readily available often at low cost. Justified and well thought out monitoring and surveil-lance strategies must be adopted which utilise just enough of the most appropriate technology. One of the first steps must be to identify avail-able technologies and understand the capability and shortcomings of each one.

4. Forms of Workplace Monitoring

The various forms of workplace monitoring that are available can be classified according to the type of technology or according to their application and are discussed by Bonsor (*n.d.*), Bryant (1995), Davies

---

[6] See www.surfcontrol.com/resources/case_studies/case_study_pace.aspx.

(*n.d.*), Marx (2002), Vorvoreanu and Botan (2000) and STOA (1999). They include:

• Telephone call and voicemail recording and logs; this may include voice and word pattern recognition;

• E-mail and Internet usage recording and logs, which may also include work pattern and web address recognition;

• Software and hardware use logging, including log-in and network usage and the detection of what is displayed on a user's screen at any given moment;

• Location tracking, for example by the use of smart cards or biometric technology to gain access to particular buildings or parts of buildings;

• Visual monitoring, for example by the use of CCTV;

• Audio monitoring *via* microphones placed in the workspace;

• Transmitters placed in vehicles for employees on the move.

Other closely related practices include genetic and HIV testing (Sayre, 1996) and even the investigation of employees' credit ratings (Quinn, 1997). Some techniques, such as genetic testing, do not necessarily qualify as electronic surveillance, but they should be a cause of concern because of their potential for producing panoptic effects (Botan and Vorvoreanu, 2000) by strengthening the control that corporations hold over their employees.

Evidence for the extent to which these various forms of surveillance are actually used by employers is provided in a survey conducted by the American Management Association (AMA, 2001). A total of 82.2% of major US firms had engaged in some form of electronic surveillance over the previous year, up from 78.4% from a similar survey conducted in 2000 and from 67% in 1999. Of those firms that admitted monitoring employees, almost half said they monitored employee phone calls, either by recording information about calls made (43.3%) or by actually listening to the calls themselves (11.9%); 46.5% stored and reviewed electronic mail and 7.8% the voicemail messages of employees. A large percentage monitored employees' computers, either by recording computer use (timed logged on, number of key strokes, time between entries, *etc.* – 18.9%), by storing and reviewing employees' computer files (36.1%), or by monitoring Internet connections (62.8%); 15.2% admitted to videotaping employee job performance and 37.7% to videotaping for security purposes. Most of these figures were an increase on those found in the previous year's survey.

5. Effects of Monitoring and Surveillance in the Workplace

Given the intrusive nature of the various forms of electronic monitoring that have been described here, concerns have been expressed about their effects on workers' privacy. The concept of 'privacy' is not easy to define and the concept of 'privacy in the workplace' perhaps even less so; if the frequently-cited Warren and Brandeis (1890) definition of privacy as the 'right to be let alone' is taken for example, it is clear that from the employer's perspective employees should not have the right to be left completely to their own devices. The employee's right to privacy will conflict with the employer's right to ensure that employees are proving effective and conforming with safety requirements and so forth.

Another way of viewing privacy that might be helpful in the workplace context is to define it as a question of control over information; privacy is jeopardised where an individual loses control over who has what information about them. Given this definition, an employee in contracting to work for an employer provides such personal data as employers are legally required to record for employment purposes and accepts certain restrictions on their freedom of movement (such as the requirement to work specified hours) in return for remuneration, access to training opportunities and so on. The question arises as to what is the level of information that an employee can reasonably expect to have to provide to their employer. Equal opportunities legislation in many countries forbids a prospective employer to make enquiries about a job applicant's marital status or childcare responsibilities, as this is irrelevant to their ability to perform the job in question. Should it be equally unacceptable for an employer to know what activities an employee is engaged in during every working hour?

The threat to privacy leads to other negative effects. For example, Clement (1992) reports that the use of electronic monitoring systems led to an increase in levels of stress, a damaging effect on workplace relationships, an emphasis on quantity rather than quality and a reduction in self-esteem with workers feeling they are not trusted. Moore (2000) points out, "We will each spend at least a quarter of our lives and a large part of our most productive years at work. This environment should be constructed to promote creative and productive activity while maintaining the zones of privacy that we all cherish." The importance of private space for employees in the workplace is not to be underestimated; in a call centre Lankshear and Mason (2001) found that, "... the availability of such private social spaces contributes to a pattern of social relations at work that make the achievement of those objectives more rather than less likely." The best 'people managers' do not need to be told that treating a person with respect will bring out the best in them.

Some studies have found that employees are disempowered by increasing levels of surveillance (for example, Sewell and Wilkinson, 1992) while others have suggested that this view underestimates workers' powers of resistance (Thompson and Ackroyd, 1995). Mason *et al.* (2002) see both of these approaches as assuming a confrontational view of workplace relationships; their studies offer a more complex view of what happens when surveillance-capable technologies are introduced. In one instance where a new computer system was 'subverted' in that it was not used in the way it was intended, this was because employees and supervisors collaborated to better meet the organisation's goals. This runs counter to the 'confrontational' model of disempowered or resisting employee vs. their would-be surveilling employer.

In another early study, Aeillo (1993) noted that the factors that influenced employees' attitudes to the introduction of electronic work monitoring include whether they participated in the design or implementation of the work monitoring system, whether and how they were informed about it and whether they understood how and why any monitoring took place. The study found that employee attitudes were dependent on the organisational climate, whether the workers were part of a cohesive work group and the quality of their relationship with their supervisor.

It may be that these and other situation-specific factors account for the apparently contradictory findings of some studies whereby in one case workers are found to be disempowered, in others to be collaborating with supervisors to meet organisational goals either actively using or in spite of the use of surveillance-capable systems. It will also be the case that in some environmental contexts such as defence industries or in medicine higher levels of surveillance/closer levels of scrutiny may be more acceptable to employees than in others. As Mason *et al.* (2002) point out, most ICT in the workplace is surveillance-capable; whether it is used for surveillance, and how, will depend on the organisational and social setting. And if it is used, how it is received by the workforce, as Aeillo (1993) suggests, will also depend on the organisational culture.

The development of surveillance-capable equipment is often driven by technologists who appear to have little knowledge of (or perhaps interest in) the human and organisational aspects of the systems for which they are responsible. In a discussion of 'awareness monitoring tools' (systems which track the presence and activities of employees to indicate their availability to interact with a geographically distant colleague), Zweig and Webster (2001) note that the computing literature promoting these systems assumes that 'availability' information is useful to enhance collaboration and performance at work. The participants in their study did not agree. Being able to be seen as physically present at their desk or workstation was not the same as being available for discussion with a colleague. Existing means of communication (for example, the telephone) were just as effective in determining whether they available for an interaction without introducing technologies that intruded on their privacy. These tools appear to be a classic case of the application of a 'hard' (technological) solution to a 'soft' (complex human and organisational) problem. Zweig and Webster note, "It appears that a technology that removes control over the type and scope of information we share with others, changes the fundamental nature of interpersonal relationships, and drives people to question their own and others' behaviours will trigger strong negative reactions." They further note that often it is the developers of these systems who evaluate them and thus fail to consider their impact on employees.

Stanton and Stam (2003) have developed this concept of the relationship between the 'triad of players': the manager, employee and the IT professional (see Figure 2). There is an exchange of resource between each of the players and a set of gains and losses associated with each of their roles. "Employees might reveal valuable information [...] in order to gain feedback useful for career growth and professional development, to gain discretionary privileges, or [...] in order to avoid job loss, financial penalties, demotion, or loss of other work-related resources."

This model is useful in highlighting the key pivotal role played by IT professionals in providing the technological means for employees to provide information and in making this information available to managers. Stanton and Stam explain that, "IT professionals might choose to enable monitoring and surveillance and provide management access to the resultant information in order to demonstrate technological mastery, support the need for staff and financial support for IT operations, and to obtain discretionary resources. On the contrary, handling and granting access to valuable information also opens up the possibility of security breaches and accompanying downtime, both of which most IT professionals wish to avoid (protective boundary closure). Additionally, any misuse of valuable information that results from IT-granted access also has the potential to be construed as an ethical breach to the extent that the IT professional facilitated it." Clearly the consequences of this power of IT professionals in terms of worker privacy, autonomy, respect and trust must be properly addressed.

Figure 2. From Stanton and Stam (2003)

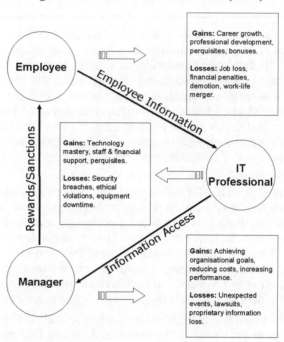

6. Social Impact Analysis

As ICT is used in practically every workplace and is by its nature surveillance-capable, almost every employee may be vulnerable to electronic monitoring and surveillance. To be seen as acceptable by employees, monitoring and surveillance need to be kept with boundaries of perceived privacy, fairness and usefulness, and not infringe psychological barriers. These boundaries may vary depending on the environment in which the organisation operates. It would seem likely that in organisations with a culture of respect for every employee, embodied in meaningful consultation and communication policies, these boundaries are more likely to be observed. On the other hand, in organisations where there is already a history of poor employee relations with a level of distrust between different groups of workers and perhaps an autocratic management approach, the introduction of surveillance-capable systems will serve to exacerbate existing divisions.

However, given the way in which ICT is continually evolving, even in the 'ideal' organisation what Sewell and Barker (2001) refer to as 'eternal vigilance' is required, "as existing forms of surveillance are moderated and give rise to new ones." The danger of leaving the development of these systems in the hands of technologists who may have little expertise nor interest in human and social issues has been noted in the previous section.

To address the issues raised here, a social impact analysis should take place before the implementation of any technology in the workplace that is surveillance-capable and then reanalysed during development and after implementation (see Figure 3). This supports the idea of negotiation and would promote good practice.

Figure 3. Social Impact Analysis Model

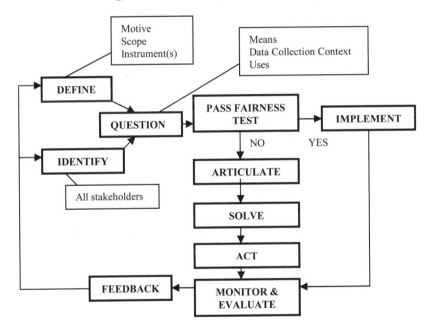

The analysis commences with a definition of the motive behind the particular workplace monitoring, the scope of the monitoring and the types of instruments envisaged. All stakeholders including both those directly and indirectly affected by the monitoring are identified. In these contexts questions are then raised regarding the specific means by which data is collected and the uses that data is and can be put to. Answers to these questions trigger concerns, issues and problems which need to be addressed and an acceptable course of action agreed. This action is monitored and evaluated and subsequently fed back into the process. In this way workplace monitoring and surveillance proposals can be properly evaluated. The reported outcome of the social impact analysis could be a test of fairness based upon the code of practice for the protection of workers' personal data (ILO, 1997) which states:

- There should be coverage for both public and private sector employees.
- Employees should have notice of data collection processes.
- Data should be collected and used lawfully and fairly.
- Employers should collect the minimum necessary data required for employment.
- Data should only be collected from the employee, absent consent.
- Data should only be used for reasons directly relevant to employment, and only for the purposes for which the data were originally collected.
- Data should be held securely.
- Workers should have access to data.
- Data should not be transferred to third parties absent consent or to comply with a legal requirement.
- Workers cannot be forced to waive their privacy rights.
- Medical data is confidential.
- Sensitive data, such as that on sex life and political and religious beliefs, should not be collected.
- Certain collection techniques, such as polygraph testing, should be prohibited.

The test of fairness would need to be passed before fair workplace monitoring could be declared and deemed to have satisfied the social impact analysis.

7. Conclusion

While there may be social benefits from a certain level of workplace monitoring and surveillance, it inevitably involves a reduction in the civil liberty of those subject to it. People do have justifiable privacy expectations even when they are in public or workspace; these expectations can be violated by monitoring and surveillance systems. Furthermore data shadows are part of our electronic persona and as such must be treated as part of us. It is unlikely that those involved in the development or deployment of surveillance-enabling technologies have considered these issues in depth. The call must be for an effective social impact analysis when such technological applications are being considered. This process should capture and take into account the opinion of those directly and indirectly affected through the use of the model previously described. Existing development practice, particularly in the early stages, would need to be amended to accommodate this process. It assumes that under appropriate conditions, employers may have a right to use workplace monitoring and surveillance systems but they also have a duty to use them responsibly. Reciprocally, those subject to legitimate surveillance may have duties (for example, not to distort the findings) as well as rights not to be subjected to some forms of surveillance or in some circumstances. By adopting the social impact approach workplace monitoring can be good practice; ignoring this process will almost certainly result in bad practice which cannot and should not be tolerated.

References

Aeillo, J. R., "Computer-Based Work Monitoring: Electronic Surveillance and Its Effects," *Journal of Applied Social Psychology*, 23 (7), 1993, 499-507.

AMA (American Management Association), *Workplace Monitoring and Surveillance: Polices and Practices*, New York, American Management Association, 2001.

Attewell, P., "Big Brother and the Sweatshop. Computer Surveillance in the Automated Office," *Sociological Theory*, 5, 1987, 87-100.

Bonsor, K., "How Workplace Surveillance Works," http://computer. howstuffworks.com/workplace-surveillance.htm [accessed 12th July 2004].

Botan, C. and McCreadie, M., "Communication, Information, and Surveillance: Separation and Control in Organisations," in J. R., Schement and Ruben B. D. (eds.), *Information and Behaviour: Vol. 4. Between Communication and Information*, New Brunswick, NJ, Transaction, 1993.

Botan, C. and Vorvoreanu, M., "What Are You Really Saying to Me? Electronic Surveillance in the Workplace," Paper presented to the Conference of the International Communication Association, Acapulco, Mexico, June 2000.

Bryant, S., "Electronic Surveillance in the Workplace," *Canadian Journal of Communication*, 20 (4), 1995, available at: http://www.wlu.ca/~wwwpress/ jrls/cjc/BackIssues/20.4/bryant.html [accessed 12th July 2004].

Clement, A., "Electronic Workplace Surveillance: Sweat-shops and Fishbowls," *The Canadian Journal of Information Science*, 17 (4), 1992, 18-45.

Davies, S., "New Techniques and Technologies of Surveillance in the Workplace," available at www.msf-itpa.org.uk/juneconf3.shtml [accessed 27th February 2001].

ILO (International Labour Organisation), *Protection of Workers Personal Data: An ILO Code of Practice*, ILO, Geneva, 1997.

Lankshear, G. and Mason, D., "Within the Panopticon? Surveillance, Privacy and the Social Relations of Work in Two Call Centres," Paper presented to the Work, Employment and Society conference, September 2001, 11-13.

Marx, G.T., "What's New about the 'New Surveillance'? Classifying for Change and Continuity," *Surveillance and Society*, 1 (1), 2002, 9-29.

Mason, D. *et al.*, "Getting Real about Surveillance and Privacy and Work," in S. Woolgar (ed.), *Virtual Society? Technology, Cyberbole, Reality*, Oxford, Oxford University Press, 2002.

Moore, A. D., "Employee Monitoring and Computer Technology: Evaluative Surveillance v. Privacy," *Business Ethics Quarterly*, 10 (3), 2002, 697-709.

Quinn, J.B., "Employers' Access to Credit Reports Unnecessary," *Indianapolis Star*, 12th March 1997, E2.

Rule, J. and Brantley, P., "Computerized Surveillance in the Workplace: Forms and Distribution," *Sociological Forum*, 7, 1992, 405-423.

Sayre, A., "Firm Withheld Results of Man's HIV Test," *Indianapolis Star*, 14th March 1996, A15.

Sewell, G. and Barker, James R., "Neither Good, nor Bad, but Dangerous: Surveillance as an Ethical Paradox," *Ethics and Information Technology*, 3, 2001, 183-196.

Sewell, G. and Wilkinson, B., "'Someone to Watch over Me': Surveillance, Discipline and the Just-in-Time Labour Process," *Sociology*, 26 (S2), 1992, 271-289.

Stanton, J. M. and Stam, K. R., "Information Technology, Privacy, and Power within Organisations: A View from Boundary Theory and Social Exchange Perspectives," *Surveillance and Society*, 1(2), 2003, 152-190.

STOA (Scientific and Technological Options Assessment), "Development of Surveillance Technology and Risk of Abuse of Economic Information," Luxembourg, European Parliament April 1999.

Tanaka, J. and Gajilan, A.T., "The Boss Is Watching," *Newsweek*, 7th July 1997.

Thompson, P. and Ackroyd, S., "All Quiet on the Workplace Front? A Critique of Recent Trends in British Industrial Sociology," *Sociology*, 29 (4), 1995, 615-633.

Vororeanu, M. and Botan, C., "Examining Electronic Surveillance in the Workplace: A Review of Theoretical Perspectives and Research Findings," paper presented to the Conference of the International Communication Association, Acapulco, Mexico, June 2000.

Warren, S. D. and Brandeis, L. D., "The Right to Privacy," *Harvard Law Review*, 5, 1890, 193-220.

Zweig, D. and Webster, J., "Where Is the Line between Benign and Invasive? An Examination of Psychological Barriers to the Acceptance of Awareness Monitoring Systems," *Journal of Organisational Behaviour*, 23, 2001, 605-633.

CHAPTER 4

Surveillance, Employment and Location

Regulating the Privacy of Mobile Workers in the Mobile Workplace

Colin BENNETT

1. Introduction

The range of complex issues embraced by the term 'privacy protection' has assumed a primary place on the political agendas of virtually every advanced industrial state. Few governmental or industry initiatives do not have some implication for the collection and processing of personal information. New practices, such as video-surveillance cameras, biometrics, smart identity cards, drug-testing, telemarketing, genetic databanks, Radio Frequency ID (RFID) and so on, can have intended and unintended consequences for the protection of personal information. Surveillance practices are changing in kind as well as degree. Thirty years ago, citizens were normally aware when personal information was being collected. Now the process of information gathering is more surreptitious. In our everyday roles as citizens, consumers, travellers, patients, students, recipients of social benefits, and employees (the subject of this paper), we continuously and unawares leave fragments of personal data behind us (Cavoukian and Tapscott, 1995).

Privacy protection in the workplace has always featured prominently in the literature on this subject. Although it is impossible to measure individuals have probably always been subjected to higher levels of monitoring and surveillance within the workplace, than without, because employers have generally asserted a greater discretion to observe the actions of "their" workers on "their" property. Of course, the tension between the manager's desire to know and the employee's right to privacy has a long history. In the 19th century employee surveillance was even regarded as a progressive method of improving worker productivity, and hence improving workers (Rule, 1996:66).

Yet the methods of workplace surveillance have changed so dramatically that they have led to more dire warnings about the corrosive effects of excessive surveillance upon the workplace environment and the rights of workers (*e.g.* Garson, 1988; Zuboff, 1988). In keeping with contemporary obsessions with reducing "risk," public and private organisations have sought corresponding mechanisms to reduce these risks when dealing with the labour market. They share human resource data on prospective employees. They require extensive medical checks, and in some cases, drug and genetic-testing. They oversee work performance through techniques such as key-stroke monitoring, and call-monitoring software. They try to detect slackers and wasters of organisational time, through video-surveillance cameras, and e-mail monitoring software. And they attempt to create a secure environment by monitoring the comings and goings of the workforce through the use of a variety of identification devices, some of which might include biometric identifiers. If a new surveillance technology has been invented, it will, to be sure, become deployed in the workplace.

The central aim of this paper is to review how the rights of the worker in the workplace have been, and can be, *regulated* in different countries under the principles and instruments of privacy protection. The first section reviews some of the key conceptual issues in order to demonstrate how the policy debates in different countries have tended to be informed by a particular definition of "information privacy" or "data protection." In the early 1970s when governments were first trying to tackle this question, certain assumptions were made about how one can, and cannot, provide a workable set of information privacy rights for citizens. These assumptions have underpinned most of the policy activity in Western societies throughout the succeeding decades and have led to a general acceptance of a set of "fair information principles" (FIPs) that appear in most international and national legal regimes. Privacy protection policy now comprises a lot more than law, however. An inventory of international, regulatory, self-regulatory and technological "policy instruments" are now at the disposal of government, business and individual citizens (Bennett and Raab, 2003). The paper then applies this framework to the range of instruments currently used to protect workplace privacy, together comprising an inventory of policy instruments designed to place some controls on the collection, processing, and disclosure of personal information by employers about employees.

This paper argues that the privacy protection issue generally, and the workplace privacy issue specifically, are undergoing a further paradigm shift as a result of the introduction of technological practices that permit a precise tracking of an individual's location and movement.[1] Organisational interests are now no longer confined to understanding individuals and their behaviours in static terms. Rather public and private agencies might have significant interests in knowing not only who we are, but also *where* we are, and how our behaviours, preferences, needs, and identities change as a result of location (*e.g.* Tuan, 1982). This shift has significant implications for the definition of the "workplace" and for the protection of "workplace privacy."

At the heart of these debates is the proliferation of the cellular (mobile) phone, and associated technologies such as Personal Digital Assistants (PDAs) and onboard vehicle telematics systems. The monitoring and tracking of movement, particularly in vehicles, is posing considerable challenges to employee privacy rights and raising a range of new and difficult questions for regulators. Under what circumstances should mobile telecommunications devices be used by employers to pinpoint an employee's location? What should happen to this data? With whom may it be shared? For what secondary purposes might it legitimately be used? The answers to these questions, however, do not lie in abandoning or revising the theory of information privacy, but to ensure that those principles are properly translated into organisational practices.

2. Information Privacy and the Fair Information Principles (FIPs)

The concept of informational privacy arose in the 1960s and 1970s at about the same time that "data protection" (derived from the German, *Datenschutz*) entered the vocabulary of European experts. The value was inextricably connected with the information processing capabilities of computers, and to the need to build protective safeguards at a time when large national data integration projects were being contemplated in different European, North American and Australasian states. These projects raised the fears of an omniscient "Big Brother" government with unprecedented surveillance power. Although concerns differed among these countries, a closely-knit group of experts coalesced, shared ideas, and generated a general consensus about the best way to solve the

---

[1] This paper is part of a larger project, funded by the National Science Foundation in the USA *(Grant No.SES-0083271),* which has attempted to gain an analytical understanding of the implementation of personal identification in geographically coded information systems, and an appreciation of the effect that identification practices have on individual privacy, sociability, trust, and risk. The co-researchers are Priscilla M. Regan, David Phillips, Michael Curry and Charles D. Raab.

problem. These efforts led to the world's first "data protection" or "information privacy" statutes (Bennett, 1992; Bennett and Raab, 2003; Bygrave, 2002; Flaherty, 1989).

The overall policy goal in every country has been to give individuals greater control of the information that is collected, stored, processed and disseminated about them by public, and in most cases, private organisations. This goal was prominent in English-speaking countries, as well as in Germany, where the concept *Informationsselbstbestimmung* (*informational self-determination*) was later developed and given constitutional status. This goal also necessitates making a distinction between the subject of the information (the data subject) and the controller of that information (the data controller). Despite some interesting debates about the application of economic, or property-based, models to give individuals greater control over "their" information (Rule and Hunter, 1999; Lessig, 1999), it has been hard to resist the conclusion that only regulatory intervention might redress the power imbalance between the data subject and the data user. Consequently information privacy has been generally defined as a problem for public policy, rather than an issue for private choice.

Once these, and other, assumptions are accepted about how one can and cannot develop public policy on privacy, a logic is set in motion that leads to a basic set of key and basic statutory principles. The historical origins of the "Fair Information Principles" (FIPs) can be briefly traced to policy analysis in Europe and the United States in the late 1960s and early 1970s (Bennett, 1992:95-115). While the codification of the principles may vary, they essentially boil down to the following tenets (Bennett and Grant, 1996:6). An organisation (public or private):

- must be *accountable* for all the personal information in its possession
- should *identify the purposes* for which the information is processed at or before the time of collection
- should only collect personal information with the *knowledge and consent* of the individual (except under specified circumstances)
- should *limit the collection* of personal information to that which is necessary for pursuing the identified purposes
- should not use or disclose personal information for purposes other than those identified, except with the consent of the individual (*the finality principle*)
- should *retain* information only as long as necessary

- should ensure that personal information is kept *accurate, complete and up-to-date*
- should protect personal information with appropriate *security safeguards*
- should be *open* about its policies and practices and maintain no secret information system
- should allow data subjects *access* to their personal information, with an ability to amend it is inaccurate, incomplete or obsolete.

These principles are, however, relative. However conceptualised, privacy is not an absolute right; it must be balanced against correlative rights and obligations to the community, although the concept of "balance" and the process of "balancing" are highly ambiguous (Raab, 1999).

Despite harmonisation there are, of course, continuing debates about how the FIPs doctrine should be translated into statutory language. There are disputes for example: about how to regulate the secondary uses of personal data – through a standard of relevance, or through specific provisions about legitimate custodians; about the limitation on collection principle and to what extent the organisation should be obliged to justify the relevance of the data for specific purposes; about the circumstances under which "express" rather than "implied" consent should be required; and about the distinction between collection, use and disclosure of information, and whether indeed these distinctions make sense or should not be subsumed under the overarching concept of "processing." How these and other statutory issues are dealt with will, of course, have profound implications for the implementation of privacy protection standards within any one jurisdiction.

The laws have also differed on the extent of organisational coverage – those in North America and Australia have historically mainly regulated public sector agencies, whereas those elsewhere (especially in Europe) encompass all organisations. This distinction is rapidly changing, however, as countries like Canada, Australia and Japan have moved to regulate private sector practices. Laws have also differed in the extent to which they regulate non-computerised files, but this distinction is also eroding. Most notably they have differed with regard to the policy instruments established for oversight and regulation (Flaherty 1989; Bennett, 1992). Most countries (with the notable exception of the United States) have set up small privacy or data protection agencies with varying oversight, advisory or regulatory powers. Some of these agencies have strong enforcement and regulatory powers; others act as more advisory *"ombudsman-like"* bodies. Some are headed by a collective commission (such as in France), others by a single "Privacy Commissioner" or "Data Protection Commissioner."

It can be finally noted that this deep and extending consensus surrounding the FIPs doctrine has occurred against a backdrop of some profound scepticism as to whether it can actually protect personal privacy and stem the inexorable tide of surveillance. Authors who have examined the issue from a broader sociological perspective have continuously raised the concern that contemporary information privacy legislation is designed to *manage* the processing of personal data, rather than to limit it. More broadly, David Lyon has contended that "the concept of privacy is inadequate to cover what is at stake in the debate over contemporary surveillance" (Lyon, 1994:196). From the perspective of those interested in understanding and curtailing excessive surveillance, the formulation of the privacy problem in terms of trying to strike the right "balance" between privacy and organisational demands for personal information hardly addresses the deeper issue. Information privacy policies may produce a fairer and more efficient use and management of personal data, but they cannot control the voracious and inherent appetite of modern organisations for more and more increasingly refined personal information (Rule *et al.*, 1980), increasingly extracted through more intrusive technologies that are altering the very boundaries between the self and the outside world.

3. From Privacy Law to Privacy Policy Instruments

Any observer of the privacy issue in the 1970s and 1980s might have concluded that the fundamental requirements of a national privacy policy were: a statutory codification of the fair information principles, an application to every public and private organisation, a coverage of all forms of personal data, regardless of sensitivity and context, and oversight and enforcement by an independent data protection agency. These conditions were generally seen as necessary and sufficient for the implementation of privacy protection policy (Bennett and Grant, 1999:7).

The privacy analysts of the 1990s and beyond, however, have questioned these assumptions and invoked the importance of other supplementary "policy instruments." A conventional wisdom emerged in the 1990s that data protection required something more than a 'one-size-fits-all' solution. According to this view, good privacy protection involves the application of several instruments, considered as a 'privacy toolkit', a 'mosaic of solutions', or a 'regulatory mix', all suggestive, but perhaps misleading, metaphors for combined approaches to data protection (Bennett and Raab: ch. 8).

Four sets of policy instruments have, at one time or another, been considered part of this "toolbox," "mosaic" or "mix." On the most general level there are a range of *international* instruments, designed to regulate the flows of personal data across national borders. The increasing ease with which personal data might be transmitted outside the borders of the country of origin has produced an interesting history of international harmonisation efforts, and a concomitant effort to regulate transborder data flows. In the 1980s, these harmonisation efforts were reflected in two international agreements, the 1981 *Guidelines from the Organisation for Economic Cooperation and Development*, and the 1981 *Convention from the Council of Europe*. In the 1990s, these efforts were extended through the 1995 *Directive on Data Protection* from the European Union which tried to harmonise European data protection law according to a higher standard of protection, and to impose that standard on any country within which personal data on European citizens might be processed. These provisions, above all, have dictated the content of the world's data protection law (Bennett and Raab, 2003: ch. 4).

A second set of *regulatory* instruments embraces the comprehensive data protection statutes, within which the fair information principles appear either explicitly or implicitly, including those in the US, Australia, New Zealand and Canada that are called 'Privacy' Acts. Data protection law has diffused rapidly around the advanced industrial world in the 1980s and 1990s, and societies more commonly characterised as "developing" are now beginning to pass similar laws. But regulation can also occur on a sectoral level, particular in the United States which has eschewed the European approach in favour of specifically targeted legislation on especially sensitive sectors (such as credit-reporting, health, and telecommunications).

A third set of instruments can be roughly described as "self-regulatory" even though the lines between regulation and self-regulation are not distinct. Within this category, we can distinguish between:

- *privacy commitments* – simple statements of policy, often appearing on websites;
- *privacy codes* – more formal and codified expressions of an organisation's or association's policy;
- *privacy standards* – which normally include procedures for independent conformity assessment; and
- *privacy seals* – the "good house-keeping seals of approval" that are awarded once an organisation has committed to, and demonstrated, an appropriate level of privacy awareness and compliance.

This typology expresses a neat cumulative logic. In practice, organisational attempts at self-regulation are more haphazard and incoherent (Bennett and Raab, 2003: ch. 6).

A final set of instruments are *technological*. Originally considered part of the "problem," information technologies can now be designed to enhance privacy protection. Technological instruments come in three forms. *Systemic instruments* are deeply embedded within the architecture of different systems; Reidenberg (1998) refers to such instruments as *"lex informatica."* *Collective instruments* are developed through central policy direction, either by the state or by large corporations. Public-key infrastructures (PKI) for service delivery are the most important examples. *Instruments of individual empowerment* require explicit choices by end-users. Examples would be the encryption, anonymising and filtering instruments commercially available for Internet users (Bennett and Raab, 2003: ch. 7).

The plurality of instruments is accompanied by a concomitant plurality of actors. Raab (1997) has discussed the co-regulation or 'co-production' of data protection, involving broader and multiple relations within and across jurisdictions, organisations and instruments. We now need to acknowledge the relevance of more actors than those who were on the privacy policy stage in the 1970s and 1980s. They include consumer organisations, the media, academics, and privacy advocates. Each of these actors is involved in the "Governance of Privacy" (Bennett and Raab, 2003). But how are these instruments and actors manifested in the context of workplace privacy?

4. Privacy Policy Instruments in the Workplace

In some respects, the fair information principles mean one thing in our role as citizens, and another in our role as workers or employees because it is difficult to assert a claim that employers have no management-related justifications for monitoring employees. They have interests in improving the efficiency and profitability of the organisation, in protecting the health and safety of workers, consumers and the public, in deterring and controlling abuse of the employment relationship, in complying with regulatory requirements, and in promoting certain public-interest considerations (Craig, 1999:26-33). The "balancing" process between an employee's right to privacy, and the employer's right to know, is inherently different from that within other organisational/individual relationships.

In the employment context, the inappropriate collection, use and disclosure of personal information can have very adverse consequences for the current and future prospects of an employee. Over and above the information privacy interests of workers, there are other privacy issues concerned with territorial privacy; even within the workplace, workers deserve some private space (in the bathroom, in the changing room, in their personal lockers). They also have certain important privacy interests over their bodies (corporeal privacy). Thus, employer claims about drug-testing, must be qualified by important limitations on the processes by which bodily fluids are extracted (Craig, 1999:18). The extraordinary and expanding scope of employee surveillance means that these "balancing" tests need to be applied with enormous sensitivity to the employment context, and to the ethics of the methods employed (Marx, 1999).

Of course, employees may already find themselves in a dependent relationship over which a long tradition of international and domestic labour law exerts an influence. Therefore, it is not simply the theory of information privacy, as outlined above, that frames the various legal and policy options. Craig (1999:53-54) demonstrates that workplace privacy is inextricably connected with competing schools of management theory. A "collective *laissez-faire* approach," for instance, discourages both legislative and judicial interference with freedom of contract, except in cases where collective representation is unlikely to yield industrial stability or justice. A "market individualism approach" asserts that state interference should be opposed, because only freedom of contract can promote the flexible environment necessary for economic growth. A "floor-of-rights approach," by contrast, supports the enactment of basic rights and standards for the benefit of candidates and employees. Clearly, if one accepts Craig's "floor-of-rights" approach, then a space is opened up for the imposition of legislative and judicial standards for workplace privacy. The other two approaches would, to differing degrees, assert that, if a worker is dissatisfied with the level of surveillance within a particular job, then she/he can always resign and seek employment elsewhere. Thus, an analysis of the policy instruments for the protection of workplace privacy is also affected by wider considerations about the appropriate role that the state should play in regulating the employee/employer relationship. And those considerations will obviously vary over time and jurisdiction.

Having said that, it is also obvious that workplace privacy rules have emerged less from pressure from unionised labour, and more from international and domestic privacy advocacy. The rules, discussed below, for the collection, processing, and disclosure of personal information in the employment context stem from the same agenda, and from the same policy community, that has produced more general instruments for privacy protection. The most general international instrument for the protection of worker privacy emerged in 1996, when the International Labour Organisation (ILO) adopted a code of practice on the protection of workers' personal data (ILO, 1997). The ILO code is now regarded as the standard among privacy advocates for protection of workers' privacy rights. The code specifies that workers' data should be collected and used consistently with Fair Information Practices (FIPs). It states that:

- There should be coverage for both public and private sector employees.
- Employees should have notice of data collection processes.
- Data should be collected and used lawfully and fairly.
- Employers should collect the minimum necessary data required for employment.
- Data should only be collected from the employee, absent consent.
- Data should only be used for reasons directly relevant to employment, and only for the purposes for which the data were originally collected.
- Data should be held securely.
- Workers should have access to data.
- Data should not be transferred to third parties absent consent or to comply with a legal requirement.
- Workers cannot be forced to waive their privacy rights.
- Medical data is confidential.
- Sensitive data, such as that on sex life and political and religious beliefs, should not be collected.
- Certain collection techniques, such as polygraph testing, should be prohibited.

The code is not binding in effect. It was intended to be used more as a template in the development of legislation, regulations, collective agreements, and work rules.

Human resources information is increasingly, however, a commodity that is transferred across national boundaries, invoking some of the other international policy instruments. Both the Council of Europe and the European Union have addressed the question of the applicability of the Treaty 108 (Council of Europe, 1981), and the Data Protection Directive (EU, 1995), respectively, to the protection of privacy in the employment context. In September 2001, the Article 29 Working Party (established under the 1995 EU Data Protection Directive) issued an influential opinion on the processing of personal data in the employment context,[2] serving to apply the words of the general Directive to the employment setting and to remind member states and employers of their obligations. The Working Party also noted that much employment-related data are highly sensitive in nature, *e.g.* union membership, sickness records, records relating to promotion, transfer, performance *etc.* and are thus prohibited from processing, unless special exemptions apply.

At the national level, many European countries, such as Austria, Germany, Norway and Sweden have strong labour codes and privacy laws which directly or indirectly restrict workplace surveillance. But most statutory rules have been developed in the context of existing national data protection legislation. Since 2000, for example, the UK Information Commissioner (formerly Data Protection Registrar) has been issuing a series of guidance codes for employer/employee relationships, including recruiting and selection procedures, records management, and monitoring at work. The Employment Practices Data Protection Code states the obligations of employers under the Data Protection Act, taking into account the requirements of the Human Rights Act 1998. Among other things, the code prohibits the making of decisions solely on the basis of automated data, requires employers to notify employees in advance of surveillance policies, requires the explicit consent of employees before sensitive data such as medical information can be collected, and places limitations on drug, alcohol, genetic, aptitude and psychometric testing within the workplace.[3] The Commissioner contends that following such practices will increase trust, encourage good housekeeping, protect organisations from legal action, and assist global businesses conform to international standards.

Most countries with established data protection regimes have, at one time or another, articulated special rules for the processing of personal data in the workplace. For example the Hong Kong Privacy Commissioner has published a Code of Practice on Human Resources Management,[4] and the Australian Commissioner has published guidelines on Internet use in the workplace.[5] Moreover, most data protection authorities will, at one time or another, have issued guidance on the use of surveillance technologies generally. Thus, statements concerning the use

---

2   Opinion 8/2001 on the Processing of Personal Data in the Employment Context.
3   Available at http://www.dataprotection.gov.uk/dpr/dpdoc.nsf.
4   Available at http://www.pco.org.hk/english/publications/listofpub.html.
5   Available at http://www.privacy.gov.au/internet/email/index.html.

of video-surveillance, the monitoring of e-mail, the use of genetic and drug-testing or biometric identifiers may have a general applicability, and make no distinction between the employment and the non-employment context. The central point is that this guidance presumes a general set of statutory rules for data protection, which all organisations are obliged to follow regardless of the context or the type of personal data being processed. The generality of some legal regimes is attributable to the difficulty of establishing when we cease to become "workers" and start becoming "citizens" or "consumers."

In Canada, a rather different regulatory framework has been established as a result of the peculiar constitutional arrangements for the federal/provincial division of powers. The 2001 privacy legislation at the federal level (the Personal Information Protection and Electronic Documents Act) only regulates the *commercial* uses of personal information; this results from the fact that the federal government could only legislate in this area under its "trade and commerce" powers within the Constitution. Employment law has always been regarded by the courts as a provincial responsibility. The extent to which employment privacy is protected in Canada is dependent, therefore, on the willingness of Canada's provinces to pass legislation, substantially similar to the federal law. So far, only Quebec, British Columbia and Alberta have passed a substantially similar provincial statutes protecting privacy in the private sector.

In the United States, there is no general data protection legislation, and therefore the rights of workers are dependent on a complex network of statutory, common law, constitutional and voluntary provisions.[6] For governmental agencies, employee privacy rights are principally governed by the long tradition of 4th Amendment jurisprudence regulating "unreasonable searches and seizures." In the private sector, however, there are few relevant statutory provisions. The Electronic Communications Privacy Act of 1986 (ECPA), which prohibits the intentional interception of electronic communications, is the only federal statute that offers workers explicit protections in communications privacy. But the ECPA contains loopholes, permitting the monitoring of phone calls and e-mail for business purposes, and allowing employers to intercept communications where there is actual or implied employee consent. There have been occasional attempts to increase workers' privacy through new legislation.[7] Post September 11th, 2001, however, the

---

[6] See the advice on workplace privacy rights given by the Privacy Rights Clearinghouse. Available at http://www.privacyrights.org/fs/fs7-work.htm.

[7] Available at http://www.epic.org/privacy/workplace.

chances of stronger privacy protection legislation passing the Unites States Congress have been slim. The passage of state legislation has also had limited success.

With respect to self-regulatory measures (commitments, codes, standards, seals), these have been developed to protect the organisational-consumer relationship in the marketplace, rather than the employer-employee relationship in the workplace. In the consumer context, these are more often genuine choices about the purchase of goods and services, and the provision of personal information. The frenzied way in which websites posted privacy policies, and subscribed to various seal programs,[8] as a way to encourage electronic commerce in the late 1990s, is testament to the important role that consumer privacy now plays in generating trust in the Internet as a medium through which goods and services can be purchased. Whether or not there is a "privacy pay-off" for those businesses that take consumer privacy seriously, as some have argued (Cavoukian and Hamilton, 2003), is still complex and controversial.

What is more clear is that public and private organisations have been far more reluctant to grant employees privacy privileges and rights in the absence of legal obligations and sanctions. A graphic illustration of the difficulty of translating self-regulatory privacy principles from the consumer to the employee context has occurred in Canada. The Canadian Bankers Association (CBA) published a code of practice for consumers in the early 1990s, revised in 1997; this code was subsequently translated into company codes by the major Canadian banks.[9] At the same time, the CBA declared that it would also develop a code for employees, one which never emerged before federal legislation was enacted in 2001. Rhetoric, therefore, about the necessity to build "employee" trust in a business or a government organisation, is less likely to convince employers voluntarily to grant rights to employees, if those rights would impinge on efficiency, profitability and other organisational values.

The same can be said for the technological policy instruments. There is no doubt that computer code can have considerable regulatory consequences in the employer-employee context (Lessig, 1999). The simple logging of cookies on a network server, for example, can be a technological decision with enormous consequences for the ability of employers to track Internet usage at work. These "systemic instruments"

---

[8]   For example http://www.truste.org and http://www.bbbonline.org.

[9]   See http://www.cba.ca.

(Bennett and Raab, 2003) or the *"lex informatica"* (Reidenberg, 1998) clearly need careful analysis in any organisational setting. And employees might voluntarily choose to use encryption of filtering instruments in order to shield their Internet activity from overly intrusive practices at work. Again, however, that choice is exercised within an employer-employee contractual relationship that may have very different consequences when exercised in the "workplace" as opposed to the home environment.

But what constitutes the "workplace"? In the concluding section, I argue that new "mobile" technologies are altering our traditional understandings of the distinction between the workplace and the non-workplace, with serious consequences for the protection of worker privacy and the application of these policy instruments.

5. The Mobile Workforce and the Mobile Worker

As Clarke (2003) notes, during the last few years "technologies have been deployed which made it increasingly feasible for large numbers of devices to be connected without being connected." Mobile technologies harbour the potential for individual surveillance and there are no doubt powerful organisations that perceive advantages for themselves in being able to locate and monitor what specific individuals are doing at specific times at specific locations. However, there is a plethora of possible relationships between the device-user and remote organisations in a "mobile" environment. As a result, as Clarke (2003) notes, "there is ample scope for people to mean different things when they use the word 'mobile'." It is, therefore, critical to any analysis of the surveillance applications and privacy implications of wireless technologies that the sense in which the term 'mobile' is being used is made explicit.

Clarke has proposed four different meanings when we talk about mobile technologies. First, devices may be 'mobile' in the limited sense of being able to be "in a different location at any given time from that in which they were at one or more previous times." Second, the term 'mobile' could mean that "a device could be anywhere, or, more carefully expressed, a device might be in any location from which transmission to another device is possible." A third interpretation of 'mobile' is in "the more substantial sense of currently moving relative to the earth's surface, but nonetheless capable of sustaining data transmission, *e.g.* as a passenger in a plane, a train, a taxi, or a car, or, less safely, as the driver of a car." A final sense of the term "is to refer to devices that are designed to be easily and conveniently portable, and to rely on wireless transmission, possibly to the extent that they do not support cable-based connections."

There are a wide variety of "mobile technologies" that are portable, that rely on wireless transmissions and that may be used to communicate from any location to another device. But none of these interrelated definitions implies *per se* that the location, less still the identity, of the user is necessarily known. This surveillance potential requires a further convergence of technology, standards-setting and organisational interests to produce what has come to be called, "location-based services" (LBS). Of course, that convergence has begun. The combination of cellular technologies, geographic positioning systems (GPS) and mapping products has produced a number of new applications designed to assist consumers, employers, parents and others "locate" individuals and objects in real time: to find the nearest retail outlet, to determine navigational coordinates, to track vulnerable people (*e.g.* children, teenagers, Alzheimer sufferers) to transmit location when 911 calls are made in times of emergency (Phillips, Regan and Bennett, 2003) and to monitor the behaviour of employees.

With regard to employee surveillance, for illustrative purposes we will focus on Clarke's third interpretation, on those "mobile" technologies that are integrated into other "mobile" technologies, *i.e.* vehicles; analysts have coined the term "telematics" to describe the collective group of technologies that enables communication, information and entertainment services delivered to motor vehicles *via* wireless technology in real-time. The industry is complex, dynamic and impossible to categorise within any degree of precision. To date, the primary values have been confined to issues of *safety* through automatic accident notification and emergency assistance functions. A second set of concerns relate to *security*, with features such as stolen vehicle tracking, remote door locking and unlocking, and remote monitoring. A third set of applications relates to *information services*; most notable are the navigation systems that provide digital maps and dynamic route guidance. A fourth, and more futuristic set of applications lies in *entertainment*, although the market for onboard devices that allow web browsing, and movie watching, has not been proven (InCode Telecom, 2001:1). Vehicles have ceased to be simply a means of transport. They have become technologies which process information about the outside world for the benefit of the driver, and can relay information about the vehicle and the driver to other agencies – law enforcement, public safety, and/or employers.

Much of the initial analysis has focused again on consumer applications, with particular attention to the feasibility of "m-commerce." There has generally been less attention paid to the employer-employee relationship. Yet, any employee with a cellular device is susceptible to having his/her actions and movements monitored whether he/she is at home, on an airplane, and of course in a company's vehicle. A variety of products are now available for the surveillance of the mobile workforce. Here are two illustrations, together with associated marketing pitches from the relevant websites.

A company called 'Fleetboss' markets a range of GPS products of varying sophistication for commercial fleet surveillance. These systems allow a GPS unit in the vehicle to read the satellite signals and record location, speed and other information. These data are transmitted to the base station automatically, which then transmits to the user's computer. The Fleetboss customised software combines mapping and vehicle data and produces customised reports on employee behaviour. It is claimed that these products can lower fuel bills, increase fleet efficiency, raise fleet productivity, control moonlighting, eliminate theft, monitor speeding, reduce accidents, identify unauthorised vehicle use, verify billing time and even be of benefit to employees. I quote:

> The Boss fleet management system "builds character" for fleet drivers who tend to drift from the desired routes and procedures of management. With The Boss system, you'll be able to see who is driving, where and when they are going and for how long. As a result, the "meeting after the meeting" is cancelled, your fuel bills go down, the excuses go away and productivity rises because side trips and non-service stops become a non-issue. With the ability to always "ride" with your drivers using The Boss fleet management system, you can monitor who, what, where and when your vehicles and tools are supposed to be used. Do you think your vehicles and tools might last longer? How much money are you losing from moonlighting? How else would you know?[10]

A second company, AirIQ, has clients that now include most of the major rental car firms in North America, owners of commercial transport fleets and service companies that operate a "mobile workforce" facilitating the dispatch of routing of calls. The AirIQ system combines five separate technologies: intelligent software systems; global positioning systems; wireless communication networks; digitised mapping software; and the Internet. AirIQ has built an intelligent messaging switch that is capable of communicating with multiple types of wireless networks and devices. Thus, the company prides itself in developing a set of solutions that are device- and wireless-agnostic.[11] Very simply, a location device (AirIQ Onboard), comprising a computer processor,

---

[10]   See http://www.fleetboss.com (accessed November 2003).
[11]   Interview AirIQ, August 16, 2002.

GPS receiver and wireless transceiver, is installed into each vehicle and keeps track of where the vehicle is (generally within 100 yards or 91,4 metres), what direction it is going, what speed it is travelling, and records and reports additional vital information. The GPS transmits data to the onboard receiver, determines a latitude and longitude "fix," and calculates the differences in fixes to determine the speed and direction of the vehicle. By pre-selecting parameters, clients choose the circumstances under which a vehicle will report. This information is then transmitted by wireless networks to the AirIQ Network Operations Center. Clients can view and access their own fleet information on digitised maps at the password protected site (www.AirIQonline.com) by using a standard Internet browser.

The corporate publicity states that "AirIQ develops mobile asset and workforce management solutions to rental vehicle fleets, commercial transport fleets and service companies... AirIQ empowers companies to manage and protect mobile resources (people and vehicles)."[12] For commercial transport fleets, customers can manage driver behaviour more effectively, locate vehicles, predict shipment arrival, inventory vehicles, provide automated maintenance reminders and retrieve lost or stolen vehicles. For service companies, the products are customised to allow fleet managers to increase efficiencies by ensuring that "the right person gets to the right place at the right time."

There are, of course, inherent limitations to onboard telematics technologies. Because these systems utilise wireless technology to communicate to and from the vehicle, the vehicle must be within cellular coverage to communicate; cellular covers approximately 95% of populated North America and some remote rural areas are still outside normal cellular coverage. Additionally, the GPS receiver must have a direct line of sight with the satellites to provide accurate location information; communication in cities with tall skyscrapers therefore poses difficulties. Nevertheless, these and other applications are currently being deployed by many companies that have an interest in managing their "mobile workforce": commercial fleet operators, taxi and limousine companies, courier and postal services, janitorial services, and so on. Potentially millions of "mobile" employees are now susceptible to more intensive and extensive surveillance, about which they may have little knowledge and control.

---

[12]   See http://www.AirIQ.com.

6. Conclusions and Implications

The literature on surveillance leaves us with the overwhelming message that the quantity and quality of surveillance have changed – both within the workplace and without. The volume of data collected and stored by both public and private organisations has facilitated a range of new practices that have developed incrementally and without much public attention or opposition. That system has developed through the uncontrolled decisions of thousands of decentralised public and private organisations, all making supposedly rational decisions that one more incremental invasion of privacy is a price worth paying for greater efficiency and/or profit. The examples cited above are supportive of David Lyon's conclusions about surveillance and the "monitoring of everyday life" (Lyon, 2001). Surveillance is "Janus-faced," according to Lyon. The same process both empowers and constrains. It gives us a variety of advantages (security, convenience, ease of communication and so on). It also enhances the power of the modern organisation to the detriment of individual privacy and to the disadvantage of marginalised groups. He demonstrates how surveillance systems have grown up to compensate for the weakening of face-to-face social relationships in which mechanisms for social integration are increasingly removed and abstract. Surveillance, then, is the necessary glue that builds trust in a "society of strangers." The "Invisible Frameworks" of integrated information and communications networks contribute to the "orchestration" of this society of strangers.

It is possible to argue that a further paradigm shift is underway with the development of mobile technologies, and associated location-based services. As these practices assume a greater importance, they become important sources of valuable information in themselves. Surveillance in turn has accommodated these changes by also becoming more mobile (Bennett and Regan, 2004). In the employment context, Lyon argues that the worker is now expected to be geographically mobile, and willing to work variable hours. "Work has become more individualised, and so have surveillance methods" (2001:40). The workplace is defined less in spatial terms (as a place where all workers have one roof over their heads), but in terms of surveillance. *You are in the workplace, where and when your activities can be monitored.* And due to the availability and relative cheapness of new surveillance methods, those occasions and places are increasingly difficult to define.

Regardless of the roots and extent of modern surveillance practices, from a political standpoint, this increase in surveillance capacity can have a dysfunctional impact on the relationship between individuals and public and private institutions. Many of these new surveillance tools are predicated on an assumption that workers cannot be trusted. Whether one is discussing video cameras, e-mail monitoring or keystroke monitoring, drug-testing, computer matching to detect fraud, or indeed, the use of Fleetboss or AirIQ, these systems serve to increase the level of distrust between individuals and the public and private organisations with which they relate. There is a circular process at work, whereby the increase in surveillance capacity reduces the level of societal trust and alienation, which in turn produces further deviant behaviour, deemed worthy of further surveillance.

But how can the theory and policies of privacy protection address these larger questions? There is a conventional wisdom amongst theorists of surveillance that they cannot. The discourse and policies of "privacy" fall far short of addressing the challenges of contemporary surveillance (Lyon, 2001; Rule *et al.*, 1980; Gandy, 1992; Marx, 1999). There are two central elements to this critique. First, privacy policy echoes rather than disturbs the classification and sorting of individuals as "disembodied abstractions." It reinforces individuation, rather than community, sociability, trust and so on. It therefore never challenges the larger questions of categorical discrimination. Moreover, privacy protection policies are "cumbersome and unresponsive" to the rapidity and diversity of technological change. At root, privacy claims tend not to see surveillance as a social question, but as a problem that can be addressed by properly implementing the fair information principles doctrine in relation to the personal data on discrete individuals.

There are, of course, larger social, economic and political issues at stake than privacy, when one considers such a complex phenomenon as the monitoring of a mobile workforce. Nonetheless, I believe the critiques of privacy protection are sometimes overstated. The modern claim to privacy does rest on a liberal notion of a boundary between the individual and other individuals, and between the individual and the state. It rests on notions of a distinction between the public and the private. It rests on the pervasive assumption that there is a civil society comprised of relatively autonomous individuals who need a modicum of privacy to make rational self-regarding choices about their lives (Bennett and Raab, 2003: ch. 1). But it also rests on the notion that social values like community, trust, sociability *etc.* are inextricably connected to the ways in which organisations collect, use, process and disclose personal information. In this sense, as Priscilla Regan has argued, society is better off when we all have greater levels of privacy (Regan, 1995:221). It is overly simple to contend that privacy is about sheltering the "sacrosanct self" behind "legal limits on the promiscuous processing of personal data" (Lyon, 2001:150).

On the question of the effectiveness of much privacy protection policy, this is, of course, dependent on context. Some privacy protection laws are indeed poorly enforced and implemented, replete with vague exemptions, and completely misunderstood by those citizens they are designed to protect. On the other hand, some are not. In some jurisdictions, stronger, unambiguous and comprehensive privacy protection laws that make no distinction between organisational sectors or the means of data processing, are overseen by activist data protection agencies that understand the range of prescriptive measures, besides legal sanction, that they can bring to bear. In some jurisdictions, a more "privacy-aware" citizenry, represented by activist privacy advocates, is far more ready to expose and critique overly intrusive surveillance practices. Although, the success of privacy protection policy is inherently difficult to measure and compare (Bennett and Raab, 2003: ch. 9), it is variable. And there are enough examples of the successful resistance to surveillance, to have a more sanguine view of efficacy of privacy protection policy, and the theory upon which it is based.

We should not downplay the importance of other modes of resistance, nor exaggerate the successes of privacy law and those who implement it. It can be argued, however, that the theory and practice of privacy protection has broadened in response to new surveillance changes in ways that are often downplayed in the sociological literature. On a conceptual level, privacy now embraces values that go beyond the interests of the possessive individual; the contemporary discourse surrounding the promotion of "trust" in new information systems is an example. Moreover, as we have seen above, privacy protection policy has broadened to encompass a plurality of policy instruments besides law, including privacy-enhancing technologies, self-regulatory tools and many mechanisms for individual empowerment.

To translate this conclusion to the practical issues raised by the monitoring of an increasingly mobile workforce, we can conclude that employee rights are far more likely to be protected where comprehensive data protection statutes, overseen by activist data protection commissioners exist. In such countries, basic privacy principles about notice, transparency, consent, relevant usage, non-disclosure, security and so on can go a long way to ensuring that only relevant information is collected on employee behaviour, and that only the appropriate people have access to that data for the right reasons. The effective implementation of privacy protection policy within an amorphous and indeterminate "workplace" will not address wider issues of workplace discrimination. Nor will it effectively interrogate and alter the changing nature of "work" in late capitalist societies. But to the extent that privacy protection policies exist, and are enforced, these wider ethical and sociological questions are certainly brought more sharply into focus.

References

Bennett, C.J., *Regulating Privacy: Data Protection and Public Policy in Europe and the United States*, Ithaca, Cornell University Press, 1992.

Bennett, C.J. and Grant R. (eds.), *Visions of Privacy: Policy Choices for the Digital Age*, Toronto, University of Toronto Press, 1999.

Bennett, C.J. and Raab, C.D., *The Governance of Privacy: Policy Instruments in Global Perspective*, Ashgate, Aldershot, 2003.

Bennett, C.J. and Regan, P., "Editorial: Surveillance and Mobilities," *Surveillance and Society*, Issue 1(4), 2004.

Bygrave, L.A., *Data Protection Law: Approaching Its Rationale, Logic and Limits*, The Hague, Kluwer International Law, 2002.

Cavoukian, A. and Tapscott, D., *Who Knows? Safeguarding Your Privacy in a Networked World*, Toronto, Random House, 1995.

Cavoukian, A. and Hamilton, T., *The Privacy-Pay-Off: How Successful Businesses Build Consumer Trust*, Toronto, McGraw-Hill, 2002.

Clarke, R., "Wireless Transmission and Mobile Technologies," 2003, at http://www.anu.edu.au/people/Roger.Clarke/EC/WMT.html.

Council of Europe, Convention for the Protection of Individuals with Regard to Automatic Processing of Personal Data (Convention 108), Council of Europe, Strasbourg, 1981.

Craig, J.D.R., *Privacy and Employment Law*, Oxford, Hart, 1999.

EU (European Union), Directive 95/46/EC of the European Parliament and of the Council on the Protection of Individuals with Regard to the Processing of Personal Data and on the Free Movement of Such Data, OJ No.L281, The EU Data Protection Directive, Brussels, 24 October 1995.

Flaherty, D.H., *Protecting Privacy in Surveillance Societies: The Federal Republic of Germany, Sweden, France, Canada, and the United States*, Chapel Hill, University of North Carolina Press, 1989.

Gandy, O., *Panoptic Sort: A Political Economy of Personal Information*, Boulder, Westview Press, 1993.

Garson, B., *The Electronic Sweatshop*, New York, Simon and Shuster, 1988.

InCode Telecom, "Telematics: How Economic and Technological Forces will Shape the Industry in the US," Incode Telecom Group, May 2001.

ILO (International Labour Organisation), *Protection of Workers Personal Data: An ILO Code of Practice*, Geneva, ILO, 1997.

Lessig, L., *Code and Other Laws of Cyberspace*, New York, Basic Books, 1999.

Lyon, D., *The Electronic Eye: The Rise of Surveillance Society*, Minneapolis, University of Minnesota Press, 1994.

Lyon, D., *Surveillance Society: Monitoring Everyday Life*, Buckingham, Open University Press, 2001.

Marx. G., "Ethics for the New Surveillance," in C. Bennett and R. Grant (eds.), *Visions of Privacy: Policy Choices for the Digital Age*, Toronto, University of Toronto Press, 1999, pp. 38-67.

OECD (Organisation for Economic Cooperation and Development), "Guidelines on the Protection of Privacy and Transborder Flows of Personal Data," OECD, Paris, 1981, at: http://www.oecd.org/dsti/sti/it/secur/prod/PRIV-EN.HTM.

Phillips, D., Regan, P. and Bennett, C., "Emergent Locations: Implementing Wireless 9-1-1 in Texas, Virginia and Ontario," in L.F. Cranor and S.S. Wildman, *Rethinking Rights and Regulations*, Cambridge, MIT Press, 2003.

Raab, C.D., "Privacy, Democracy, Information," in B. Loader (ed.), *The Governance of Cyberspace*, London, Routledge, 1997, pp. 155-74.

Raab, C.D., "From Balancing to Steering: New Directions for Data Protection," in C. Bennett and R. Grant (eds.), *Visions of Privacy: Policy Choices for the Digital Age*, Toronto, University of Toronto Press, 1999, pp. 68-93.

Regan, P.M., *Legislating Privacy: Technology, Social Values and Public Policy*, Chapel Hill, University of North Carolina Press, 1995.

Reidenberg, J., "Lex Informatica: The Formulation of Information Policy Rules Through Technology," *Texas Law Review*, Vol. 76, 1998, pp. 552-593.

Rule, J., MacAdam, D., Stearns, L. and Uglow, D., *The Politics of Privacy: Planning for Personal Data Systems as Powerful Technologies*, New York, Elsevier, 1980.

Rule, J., "High-Tech Workplace Surveillance: What's Really New?," in D. Lyon and E. Zureik (eds.). *Computers, Surveillance and Privacy*, Minneapolis, Minnesota University Press, 1996.

Rule, J. and Hunter, L., "Towards Property Rights in Personal Data," in C. Bennett and R. Grant (eds.), *Visions of Privacy: Policy Choices for the Digital Age*, University of Toronto, Toronto Press, 1999, pp. 168-81.

Tuan, Y-F., *Segmented Worlds and Self: Group Life and Individual Consciousness*, Minneapolis, University of Minnesota Press, 1982.

Zuboff, S., *In the Age of the Smart Machine: The Future of Work and Power*, New York, Basic Books, 1998.

PART III

ETHICAL ANALYSIS

CHAPTER 5

The Importance
of Workplace Privacy

Philip BREY

1. Introduction

Existing discussions of privacy, including discussions of workplace privacy, too often rely on a vague and broad notion of privacy that cannot properly informed detailed analyses of specific privacy issues. As a result, such analyses often rely heavily on *ad hoc* considerations and intuitions, and analyses of different privacy issues do not add up to a coherent view on privacy. What is still lacking in the privacy literature is an adequate operationalised notion of privacy that affords a distinction between different types of private affairs, privacy rights, and privacy intrusions. In this paper, I attempt to develop such an operationalised notion of privacy and apply it to the analysis of workplace privacy issues. In section 2, I present this operationalised conception of privacy, which I then use in section 3 to identify the main privacy issues in today's workplace. In section 4, I identify the most important privacy rights in the workplace, and consider arguments for and against restrictions to these rights based on the employer's interest in good work performance. I summarise my main conclusions in section 5.

2. Towards an Operationalised Notion of Privacy

Privacy as Limited Access to Personal Affairs

Systematic study of the notion of privacy began with Warren and Brandeis' famous essay titled "The Right to Privacy" (1890), in which privacy is defined as "the right to be left alone." Since then, countless other definitions of privacy have been presented, many in the context of elaborate theories of privacy, that try to get at the core of this abstract and slippery notion. Theories of privacy generally allude to privacy as a right of persons that is to provide protection against interference by third

97

parties into their private affairs. In many theories, this right to non-interference is defined in terms of access and control: privacy rights are to restrict access to private affairs and give those persons whose private affairs are at issue the exclusive right to control such access.

Some authors have introduced the notions of "information" or "knowledge" as a defining feature of privacy (Westin, 1967; Fried, 1986; Parent, 1983). In such information-based conceptions of privacy, privacy is defined in terms of restrictions on access to, or control over, personal information, and intrusions on privacy are defined as situations in which personal information is collected or disseminated without consent of the individual who is the topic of this information. However, while it appears that many privacy issues revolve around the use of personal information, information-based conceptions of privacy are clearly flawed, as there is a number of privacy issues that cannot be fitted into an informational mold. That is, there are types of actions that can be recognised as intrusions on privacy but that do not seem to centrally revolve around the collection or dissemination of personal information.

Specifically, there are various sorts of intrusions into private affairs in which the violation of privacy seems to consist on the fact that these affairs are disturbed or disrupted, rather than that information is acquired about them. For instance, unlawful entry or trespassing, which is sometimes described as the violation of the privacy of someone's home, does not seem to revolve around information collection. Such an event may perhaps result in the collection of personal information by the intruder (if the intruder is not blind), but the violation of privacy does not seem to centrally reside in this collection but rather in the disturbance of private affairs. Likewise, not keeping a certain distance when talking to someone or sitting or standing next to them or touching their body may also be construed as violations of privacy even though they do not centrally involve the acquisition of personal information.

Therefore, if privacy is defined in terms of (control over) access, then clearly it is not just informational or cognitive access that is involved but also physical access, as when someone creates disturbances in private affairs. This corresponds well with Warren and Brandeis' description of the right to privacy as the right to be left alone: it is not just the right to be left alone from the gaze or opinions of others, but also the right to control physical interference by others into one's private affairs. Adhering to the notions of access of control we may, with Ferdinand Schoeman, say that "a person has privacy to the extent that others have limited access to information about him, limited access to the intimacies of his life, or limited access to his thoughts or his body"

(Schoeman, 1984:3). The right to privacy is then the right of persons to control such access to their personal affairs.

Cognitive Access, Physical Access and Informed Control

So far, I have distinguished two forms of access to private affairs: *cognitive access*, which is access to information about private affairs of a person, either through direct observation or through indirect means, and *physical access*, which involves direct interventions into private affairs that create a disturbance in them. In discussing cognitive access, I have stated that such access may result in the collection or dissemination of information. Privacy violations that involve the collection of information about private affairs may be called *snooping*, and those that involve the dissemination of such information may be called *exposure*. In snooping a third party makes personal information available to herself, whereas in exposure she makes it available to other parties. Cognitive access may moreover take various forms, depending on how information is collected. Cognitive access may involve live, unaided observation of private affairs, mediated observation through a camera or telephone line), or access to separate bearers of personal information *e.g.* electronic databases, paper documents, photographs.

Physical intrusions, in which privacy is violated through physical interventions, may also be called *disturbances*. The term "physical intrusion" is meant in a broad sense here, to include physical interruptions of events, disturbances that take place by talking or making noise and disturbances that occur in virtual environments; when someone breaks into a private chat-room and starts insulting the participants, I would also call this a physical intrusion. Obviously, there are many privacy violations in which cognitive and physical intrusions occur jointly. This is only logical, because while disturbing the intruder usually also perceives things that are private (unless the person that creates the disturbance is blind and deaf).

There are also privacy violations that do not just centre on cognitive access (snooping or exposure) or physical access (disturbance). Take, for example, a landlord who has installed cameras in the apartments of his tenants, and who does not just observe these tenants in their everyday affairs, but also makes systematic use of his observations to control the behaviour of his tenants. If, for instance, he sees a tenant breaking house rules in their apartments, he may coerce her into obeying them in the future, or punish her by temporarily cutting of her electricity or by evicting her. This landlord is not necessarily creating a disturbance (because he may never enter any of the apartments) nor is he just snooping. Rather, he is making systematic use of his cognitive access to his tenant's apartments to control their behaviour and living circumstances.

I would call this type of privacy intrusion "surveillance," were it not that this term is ambiguous; in a broad sense, systematic observation of subjects that does not result in direct attempts to control the thoughts and behaviour of these subject is sometimes also called surveillance. So I opt instead for informed control. What is essential about informed control is the ability of a third party to exercise control over a person through his knowledge of private affairs of that person. This control may either be confined to the private affair about which the third party knows, or it may (also) affect other aspect of the person's life. For instance, if the snooping landlord observes that a tenant uses illegal substances, he may coerce her into stopping this behaviour or doing it less frequently, but he may also use this information to blackmail the tenant, without necessarily interfering with the drug use itself. In the first instance, there is informed control over an observed private affair in that the conditions under which the private affair takes place are controlled. In the second instance, there is control over broader aspects of a person's life based on knowledge of a private affair. Notice, moreover, that informed control *may* include physical intrusions on privacy (when the landlord walks into an apartment every time he observes that rules are broken), but they are not *required*.

To summarise, privacy intrusions come in three kinds:

(1) unauthorised cognitive access (snooping and exposure)

(2) unauthorised physical access (disturbances)

(3) informed control (control over a private affair or broader aspects of a person's life).

Types of Private Affairs

So far, I have defined privacy in terms of limited access to private affairs, and I have described three modes of access to private affairs and corresponding ways in which privacy can be intruded on. I have not, however, said much about the objects of such access or intrusion: *private affairs*. What is a private affair, and what kinds are there? I will define private affairs as things connected to one's private life or work that one considers to be private. It turns out that there are many different kinds of private affairs. Private affairs may include behaviours, information bearers, aspects of the body, private rooms, personal objects and social events. Corresponding to these different types of private affairs are different types of intrusions on privacy. For example, violating the privacy of a social event like a dinner party (whether through cognitive

100

access, physical access or informed control) is different from violating so-called informational privacy through access to personal information, which is again qualitatively different from violating privacy by going through the contents of someone's purse.

There have been few attempts in the privacy literature to systematically distinguish different kinds of private affairs and relate these to a theory of privacy. Westin (1967) has made a distinction between informational and relational privacy, where relational privacy is the right to determine one's own personal relationships and conduct without other people observing and interfering with them, and informational privacy is the right to selective disclosure of personal data. The private affairs corresponding to these two types of privacy are personal relationships and conduct, and personal data and their bearers. Nouwt and Vorselaars (in Bekkers *et al.*, 1999) have further introduced the category of physical privacy, to supplement the notions of relational and informational privacy. Physical privacy is the right to control access to one's body; the private affairs it relates to are aspects of one's body. Allen (1999) also introduces a notion of physical privacy, but defines it more broadly to include both bodily integrity and restricted access to the home and one's personal belongings.

I believe that these attempts to define different types of privacy in relation to different types of private affairs should be further refined. Westin's and Nouwt and Vorselaars' notion of relational privacy lumps together personal relationships and individual conduct, which are really distinct categories. I therefore propose to distinguish them: one type of private affair consists of individual conduct *e.g.*, things one does when alone at home and another consists of personal relationships, or social conduct involving instances of private communication and social interaction. Likewise, Allen correctly defines physical privacy to not only include bodily integrity but also integrity of the home and personal belongings. But then it also makes sense to distinguish the two: the human body is one type of private affair, and personal spaces and objects constitute another type, and different types of privacy rights apply to each of them.

Consequently, we may distinguish five basic kinds of private affairs, with corresponding rights to privacy: (i) the human body; (ii) personal spaces and objects; (iii) bearers of personal information; (iv) individual conduct and (v) social conduct. I will discuss these now in turn.

(i) The Human Body

By the human body, I mean the physical or biological body, with all its unique features as they apply to a specific person. Such unique features include physical and biochemical properties such as height, weight, facial characteristics, visual features of the nude body, fingerprints, medical conditions, the biochemical composition of blood, urine and feces and genetic make-up. Many such aspects of the body are privacy-sensitive, although there is often significant variation in the degree to which people hold certain aspects of their body to be private. This variation is strongly conditioned by culture, religion and gender. For example, in traditional Islamic cultures the female face is considered to be a private affair and is hidden in public areas, while in many non-western cultures, the nude body is not very privacy-sensitive, and public displays of nudity may be acceptable.

The human body is increasingly a contested site, as employers, law enforcers and others increasingly seek access to aspects of the body. Unwanted cognitive access may involve observation with the naked eye, mediated observation *e.g.*, through camera observation or body scans, medical tests, genetic tests, drug tests and biometric registration (recordings of fingerprints, iris prints and face-prints). Such cognitive access may be used for various types of informed control, including an amount of control over the composition and appearance of the body and over biological functions. Unwanted physical access may include invasion of body space, unwanted touch, unwanted medical examinations and drug tests, unwanted registration of biometric properties like fingerprints, body searches, cavity searches, sexual assault and rape.

(ii) Personal Spaces and Objects

Personal spaces include the home, other personally owned and used spaces like the confines of one's car, and rented or appropriated personal spaces like a private chat-room on the Internet or a claimed picnic spot. Personal objects are objects owned, hired or appropriated by a person for his or her personal use, such as jewellery, vacuum cleaners, refrigerators, teddy bears, *etc.* The privacy-sensitivity of personal objects or belongings may differ a great deal: mundane objects like pencils and vacuum cleaners will rarely be considered privacy-sensitive, whereas potentially revealing or embarrassing items like teddy bears, sexual apparel and antidepressants may be highly privacy-sensitive. Still, people sometimes want to keep mundane objects at their homes private as well, since these may still provide a lot of information about their personal lives.

102

Personal spaces and objects may be the subject of unauthorised cognitive and physical access in various ways: through house searches, break-ins, seizures, camera surveillance, remote sensing and ordinary peeking and snooping by curious third parties like house guests and fellow employees who cannot keep themselves from going through someone's personal belongings.

(iii) Bearers of Personal Information

Bearers of personal information are media that contain information about aspects of a person, for instance about her individual conduct, her thoughts and beliefs, her personal relations, aspects of her body or her personal belongings. Such bearers may include files, paper records, personal notes, pictures, diaries, electronic databases, video tapes, CD-Rs, personal digital assistants (PDIs), *etc.* They may encode information in various forms, including linguistic, numerical and pictorial, and may include video and audio recordings. Bearers of personal information may be owned or used by the person in question. If so, they are a special type of personal object (as defined in the previous paragraph). However, many bearers of personal information are not owned and used by the subject of the information but by third parties, including doctors, insurance companies, banks, employers, government institutions, media agencies, internet providers, supermarkets and so on.

Bearers of personal information may be the subject of unauthorised physical access, resulting in disturbances if they are mishandled, but it is their cognitive function that is most important here: cognitive access to them may also provide cognitive access to aspects of someone's private life, and may offer concomitant possibilities for informed control.

(iv) Individual Conduct

Individual conduct is defined in the context of this paper as non-social conduct, being individual behaviour that does not (centrally) include interactions with others. A particularly important type of individual conduct from a privacy point of view is *solitary behaviour*, being behaviour that one performs when one is alone or "by oneself," without companions or observers that are believed to have access to one's behaviour. Solitary behaviour is often very privacy-sensitive. It may include behaviours that are quite similar to ones performed in more social or public settings *e.g.*, reading, watching TV, working but also involves all kinds of intimate behaviours *e.g.*, taking care of bodily functions, autoeroticism, behaviours that do not adhere to normal public standards *e.g.* laziness, sloppiness, gluttony, wearing outrageous combinations of clothing, exercising private personal hobbies, self-experimentation *e.g.*, making faces in front of a mirror, and generally, performing all kinds of actions that one would not normally perform in public, or even in a relatively intimate setting with family or friends.

Individual conduct, including solitary behaviour, is increasingly subjected to monitoring *i.e.*, cognitive access, particularly through camera surveillance and increased electronic registration of behaviour *e.g.*, purchases, money withdrawals, vehicle use, computer use, Internet use.

(v) Social Conduct

Next to individual behaviour there is social behaviour: interactions with other human beings, whether they involve playing pool, making love, working together to plant a tree, having an e-mail exchange, or having a chat about the weather. From a privacy point of view, social behaviour deserves to be treated separately from individual or non-social behaviour, both because of special privacy considerations that apply to (solitary) individual behaviour and because of special privacy considerations for social behaviour, that result from the fact that it includes shared intimacy and trust. Indeed, many social interactions are private to some degree in that they are not meant to be (closely) observed or intruded on by third parties. One important form of social interaction that deserves special mention is *verbal communication*. Verbal communication, whether face-to-face, over the telephone, or *via* e-mail, SMS or Internet chat, is often considered private, either because it contains privacy-sensitive information or because the conversationalists seek seclusion so as to create intimacy, trust or confidentiality between them.

Like individual conduct, social conduct is increasingly subjected to monitoring, particularly through camera surveillance and increased electronic monitoring of (technologically mediated) social interactions, for instance through telephone and e-mail monitoring.

In summary, I have argued that privacy can be defined in terms of the right of persons to control access to their personal affairs. I have argued that three types of access must be distinguished in the context of this definition: cognitive access (snooping and peeking), physical access (disturbances) and informed control (control, by means of cognitive access, over a private affair or broader aspects of a person's life). I have also argued that privacy rights must be specified in the context of five distinct types of (potentially) private affairs: aspects of the human body, personal spaces and objects, bearers of personal information, individual conduct and social conduct (including, centrally, verbal communication).

3. Privacy Issues in the Workplace

As stated in the introduction, workplace privacy is increasingly a contested issue in organisations. Many new methods of monitoring workers have been developed in recent decades, building particularly on new developments in information technology and medical technology. In this section, I will outline the main privacy issues that play in today's workplace. I will do this in the context of my previous operational analysis of the concept of privacy. My typologies of private affairs and privacy intrusions are helpful in defining and categorising challenges to workplace privacy, particularly challenges induced by new technologies. I will take as my point of departure the five types of potentially private affairs outlined in the previous section, and I will ask to what extent they appear in the workplace as contested objects. In doing so, I will take account of the fact that privacy intrusions in the workplace may take the form of unauthorised cognitive or physical access or informed control.

A. The Human Body in the Workplace

Worker's bodies are increasingly the subject of scrutiny by employers. From genetic dispositions to fingerprints, from the presence of scar tissue on the lower abdomen to the presence of alcohol traces in worker's urine, employers increasingly know about, or are able to find out about, aspects of their worker's bodies. In some professions, moreover, such monitoring is accompanied by routine physical interventions, like periodical medical and drug tests and body scans. In an increasingly competitive business climate, employers are bent to know whether workers have medical conditions of genetic dispositions that may impact their work, or whether workers have a substance abuse problem. Also, organisations increasingly use biometric authentication and verification methods to provide security, which also touch on aspects of their worker's bodies. A wide variety of new and improved technologies has been instrumental in allowing employers access to aspects of their employee's bodies, and legislation has often not kept up with them.

Some of the main workplace privacy issues in relation to worker's bodies are the following:

Medical Tests and Medical Background Checks

Employers increasingly make use of medical tests and access to existing medical records to assess the health of their employees. Psychological assessments are also increasingly sought. Such medical information increasingly plays a role in hiring and firing decisions, work benefits and career development, and its use is therefore controversial (Simms, 1994; Humber and Almeder, 2001; Rosenberg, 1999).

Drug Testing

Some employers routinely test their employees for substance abuse. Such tests are not normally defined as medical tests, and its use is more controversial that medical tests (Cranford, 1998; Gilliom, 1994; Rosenberg, 1999).

Genetic Testing

Genetic testing is usually performed for medical reasons, to determine whether a (prospective) employee is genetically predisposed to develop certain medical conditions, like cancer and hepatitis. Genetic tests are hence not ordinary medical tests, because the subject may not have any medical conditions, and the conditions for which he or she is tested positively may never actually develop. Their use is controversial, because they are not always reliable and the (prospective) employee may never actually develop a disease for which there is a genetic predisposition (Long, 1999; Chadwick *et al.*, 1999).

"Pat down" Searches and X-ray Body Scans

In professions with high security risks, employees may be routinely subjected to "pat down" searches, some of which may also require (partial) undressing or even cavity searches, and to X-ray body scans. In an X-ray body scan, a technology used mainly at airports, low-dose X-rays are used to see beneath a person's clothing and undergarments. The result is an image of a nude body, with any devices or foreign objects that may be carried on the body. Major personal details of bodies, such as the size and shape of breasts and genitals, mastectomies, catheter tubes and penile implants, are revealed in such images (Murphy and Wilds, 2001). This technology is usually used with the consent of the person whose body is scanned but can also be used – and is being used – secretly.

Biometric Screening

Biometrics methods are increasingly used in the workplace as authentication and verification devices, for instance to monitor access to a building or area, to keep time on workers, or to monitor access to computer systems. Common biometric methods include iris scans, face scans and thumbprints. Biometric screening involves the electronic storage of privacy-sensitive biometric information, as well as the scanning process itself, which is experienced by some as privacy-intrusive (see Hes,

Hooghiemstra and Borking, 1999; Alterman, 2003; Van der Ploeg, 2003).

Camera surveillance

In most cases, camera surveillance in the workplace will not reveal private information about bodies or bodily conditions. Yet, it sometimes does so, for example if used in areas where employees (partially) undress or take care of their body. Camera surveillance in the workplace increasingly takes place in more (*semi-*) private environments, like offices, restrooms and leisure areas, and has been argued to invade privacy (McCahill and Norris, 1999; Dubbeld, 2003).

In most cases where bodily privacy is at issue in the workplace, it is cognitive access that is involved, which may in turn result in informed control (over the employee's drug use, health care, career development, *etc.*). Physical access to worker's bodies is not gained often, and is usually limited to medical or drug tests and body searches. (In stating this, I am not considering unwanted intimacies, which of course do occur often in workplaces. I am only considering physical intrusions on privacy that happen as a matter of company policy.)

B. Personal Spaces and Objects in the Workplace

Workers frequently bring personal belongings with them to the workplace. These may include pens, wallets, handbags, personal digital assistants, laptops, plants, framed pictures of the family, and so on. Handbags and desk drawers may contain personal items like cosmetics, personal address books, medication and feminine hygiene products. Workers may also use the workplace as a temporary storage space, for example for groceries and other personal belongings. Workers also frequently have a workspace for their personal use (*e.g.* an office space) and personal equipment, furniture or tools (*e.g.*, a desk, a personal computer, a closet) that they come to use as they own, and that they come to control. Workers often end up personalising their workspace, not only by bringing in their own personal belongings, but also by modifying company property, for example by rearranging furniture or by choosing screensavers, backgrounds and settings on their PC. Workers tend to have privacy expectations concerning the access by others to personal belongings brought to work, and often also have an expectation of privacy regarding their workspace, *e.g.*, the expectation that no one enters their office unannounced or goes through the contents of their filing cabinets or computer hard drive without their consent. Naturally, going through personal items like a handbag will be considered a greater violation of privacy than scrutinising someone's tools or office furniture.

Privacy issues that may come up in relation to personal spaces and objects in the workplace may include unauthorised access by employers and fellow-workers to someone's personal workspace, camera surveillance of workplaces, workplace searches, and surveillance or searches of the contents of PCs. Workplace searches may include searches of employee offices, desks, lockers, personal items like purses and gym bags, files and mail. Surveillance and searches of the contents of PCs may involve inspecting the software and files on the employers' PC and taking random "snapshots" of the PC's desktop. In many professions, the working environment is increasingly a PC environment. The virtual work environment of a PC is much easier to inspect than a physical work environment, because it is usually possible for employers and system operators to have remote access to it, and because it is possible to perform quick searches for specific items.

C. Bearers of Personal Information in the Workplace

A number of privacy issues in the workplace concern access to media that contain personal information about employees. Some such media may be in the possession of employees themselves, like personal belongings brought to work by workers that contain personal information (diaries, personal address books, photo albums) or items with personal information that were produced or received by the employee while at work *e.g.*, personal e-mail, paychecks, internet cookies. Searches of employee's belongings and surveillance of workplaces and electronic work environments may result in employers learning about such private information.

Other media may not be in possession of the employee herself but may be owned by (various departments in) the organisation, or be found outside the organisation but still be obtainable by its management. Regarding the body, medical records have already been mentioned as one type of medium of this sort. Many more personal records and media may be found in organisations, including financial records, personnel files, minutes of meetings, video surveillance tapes, and so on. Such files are usually meant to be accessible to a limited number of people, and it would be considered a breach of privacy if other persons in the organisation were granted access as well.

Organisations also often perform *background checks* on prospective employees, which are increasingly easy to perform through the rise of the Internet and electronic databases. Employees may, depending on legal limitations that may apply, check address history, criminal background, civil background, driving history, credit reports, and past employment. Obviously there are many employees who would consider at least some of these checks, when performed without their consent, a violation of their privacy.

D. *Individual Conduct in the Workplace*

Individual conduct in the workplace may either consist of working behaviour (*e.g.*, typing, drawing, soldering) or behaviour for personal maintenance and leisure, *e.g.* snacking, reading internet newspapers, visiting the toilet, grooming, listening to music. Working behaviour and personal maintenance and leisure of course sometimes mix, as when someone is working while listening to music or eating. The expectations of privacy for these three types of behaviour will depend on the attitudes and beliefs of the worker, the setting in which work takes place, and previous agreements that have been made. Obviously, surveillance cameras in a toilet will generally be considered unacceptable, whereas keystroke registration may be considered acceptable if it is part of an agreement between employer and employee.

Privacy issues that may play in relation to individual conduct in the workplace include unauthorised access by employers and fellow-workers to a private or temporarily privatised space in which someone is engaging in private behaviour, *e.g.*, a toilet or an office with a do-not-disturb sign, camera surveillance, computer keystroke monitoring, internet website monitoring, behaviour monitoring using smart badges and motion detectors, *e.g.* to check if an employee washes hands after using the bathroom, location tracking using electronic employee badges, and satellite tracking (Givens, 2001). Camera surveillance and PC and Internet monitoring are arguably the two most powerful techniques for monitoring individual conduct. Camera surveillance theoretically makes it possible to record and observe an employer's each and every movement. The monitoring of PC and internet use by their employees can give employers detailed, complete information on what workers type, read, access or download when working on their PC (see Ball, 2001; Wood, 1998; Alder, 1998; Brey, 1999; Rosenberg, 1999).

E. *Social Conduct in the Workplace*

Social conduct in the workplace may, like individual conduct, be either work-related (*e.g.*, teamwork, staff meetings) or directed at personal maintenance or leisure (*e.g.*, joint lunches, social chats). Mixes occur as well, as when a conversation combines personal and work-related elements. Obviously, social conduct directed at personal maintenance or leisure will generally be more privacy-sensitive than social interactions that are work-related. However, work-related social interactions may also have a private character, involving confidentiality and trust, as when problems at work are a topic of discussion, or more generally when those who are interacting have an expectation of privacy.

As noted earlier, social interactions between persons may occur in unmediated form ("face-to-face" or in person) or be technologically mediated (*e.g.*, telephone, e-mail, internet chat, SMS, voice mail, computer-supported collaborative work). Many privacy issues that apply to individual conduct in the workplace apply to social conduct as well. Other privacy issues are uniquely associated with social conduct. These include, amongst others, issues involving the monitoring of communications, as in telephone monitoring and e-mail monitoring. Another important privacy-related element in social interaction is, as previously mentioned, the potential importance of confidentiality, trust and intimacy between persons, for example between an employee and a fellow-worker or client, that may be violated by monitoring.

4. Workplace Privacy and Employer's Interests

In most discussions of workplace privacy, it is recognised that employees have legitimate claims to privacy rights at work. In most discussion, however, it is held that such rights are to be balanced against the rights or interests of employers and other parties, which may require limitations on these privacy rights. In what follows, I will first make the case, based on the discussion of workplace privacy issues in the preceding section, that employees have legitimate expectations of privacy even while at work. I will argue that the privacy issues outlined in the previous section point to a set of *prima facie* privacy rights for employees that ought to be limited only if there are good reasons to do so. I will then consider some of the main arguments that have been made for restrictions on workplace privacy, which usually allude to the employer's interest in good work performance by his employees. I will then consider weaknesses in these arguments for restrictions on workplace privacy, and argue that they do not succeed in justifying strong curtailments of privacy rights at work in most circumstances.

Prima Facie *Privacy Rights in the Workplace*

In discussing privacy in the workplace, it may be useful to distinguish between privacy rights that hold in principle and privacy rights that hold in practice, *i.e.* after calibration with circumstantial factors which may include other rights or interests. In general, rights of any kind may have to be weighed against other rights or they may be voluntarily forfeited, so that rights that are held in principle may not turn out to hold in practice. For instance, people may have a right to smoke, but it can be justifiably argued that this right may not be exercised in confined public areas because it collides with other people's rights to clean air, or in clean rooms because it could damage private property. I therefore want to arrive at a conception of the principled or *prima facie* privacy rights of employees, that may be argued to hold in advance of any balancing of such rights against other rights or interests, and preceding any possible voluntary forfeitures of such rights. On the basis of such principled privacy rights in the workplace, we may then go on to ask under what circumstances curtailments of such rights can be justified.

A determination of *prima facie* privacy rights in the workplace should ideally be sought through a method of reflexive equilibrium (Van den Hoven, 1997) in which existing privacy theory is balanced against privacy intuitions, existing social norms and practices, empirical research on the psychological and social dimensions of privacy, and other relevant data. I will not perform a full analysis of this kind here, but take a bit of a shortcut, relying mainly on existing privacy norms, laws and intuitions to arrive at a set of *prima facie* privacy rights in the workplace. I propose that *prima facie* privacy rights apply to a thing or activity in the workplace (*e.g.*, the use of a toilet, an e-mail message, the contents of a purse) when such things or activities are generally considered to be private outside the workplace. More precisely:

> *Prima facie* privacy rights apply to an entity (thing or activity) in the workplace if and only if entities of that type outside the workplace are generally considered to be private affairs.

In the discussion of privacy issues in the workplace in the previous section, I have already identified many issues involving affairs that at least some people claim to be private. In some cases, this may involves entities that may also be contested outside the workplace as to whether they should be considered private. This may happen either because there are no shared social norms on whether or to what extent an entity should be considered private and therefore subject to privacy rights (*e.g.*, some cultures or traditions consider the female face to be private, whereas most others do not), or because the private nature of a type of entity is heavily dependent on situational factors and subjective intentions (*e.g.*, whether a conversation is private depends in part on the intentions of the talkers and on the setting in which they choose to have their conversation).

For most of the privacy issues identified in the previous section, however, I believe that general agreement exists that the entities in question are private in ordinary circumstances. The disagreement about

111

them concerns the extent to which the special circumstances of a work-place setting can void these ordinary privacy rights. At least the following matters considered in the previous section would be considered private to some degree in ordinary circumstances:

- aspects of the human body that are not visible in everyday life
- the contents of purses, shopping bags, desk drawers and lockers
- rooms that function as a working or living environment for a person or group of persons
- solitary forms of behaviour like toilet visits and solitary work breaks
- conversations about personal or leisure subjects
- person-to-person postal, voice mail or e-mail messages
- files or records with personal information.

Prima facie privacy rights apply less obviously to activities that are strongly work-related and that involve few personal elements, such as many individual working activities and work-related interactions and conversations. This is because these activities often do not include many privacy-sensitive aspects like personal information, intimacy or confidentiality. However, a case can be made that such activities are still subject to some privacy rights. Helen Nissenbaum has argued in an important paper that even though there is a diminished expectation of privacy in public places, people still have justifiable privacy expectations even when they are in public (Nissenbaum, 1998). Her argument is that surveillance in public places that involves the electronic collection, storage and analysis of information on a large scale, without the consent of the public, violates privacy because this practice does not conform to normal information-governing norms in public places. Such norms require that observers or information collectors make themselves known and do their work visibly (*e.g.*, surveilling police officers) and maintain contextual integrity, meaning that information deemed appropriate in one context is not used in contexts for which it was not intended and for which it was not voluntarily made available. Such contextual integrity is often not maintained in electronic surveillance, because the information may easily be used in different contexts.

Nissenbaum's argument seems to apply to the workplace as well as it does to public areas. Here, solitary working activity and work-related interactions and conversations are not usually privacy-sensitive to the extent that accidental or intentional intrusions on them by third parties necessarily constitute serious violations of privacy, but sustained intense surveillance of such activities, possibly even done in secret and possibly

112

performed without accountability for the use of the information thus collected, appears to run contrary to normal information-governing norms and normal expectations of contextual integrity, and can therefore be identified as *prima facie* violations of privacy. These violations of privacy clearly do not just rest on cognitive access of the surveillor to working activity of employees, but also on the informed control that such cognitive access affords, which may result, next to diminished workplace privacy, in diminished worker autonomy, the erosion of trust between employee and employer, lower morale, and stress and health problems (Persson and Hansson, 2003; Brown, 2000; Brey, 1999).

I conclude, then, that *prima facie* workplace privacy rights apply, to a lesser or greater degree, to nearly all the contested items that were discussed in the previous section.

Arguments for Restrictions on Workplace Privacy

The main argument that has been put forth in favour of a limited right to privacy in the workplace is that employers have a strong, legitimate interest in monitoring the performance of their employees, and that this strong interest cannot be reconciled with strong privacy rights for employees. Good performance here relates to more than the question of whether employees work hard enough, create enough work output or create output that has enough quality. Good performance also means not harming the organisation (for example though carelessness, wastefulness, theft and embezzlement, or through baseless lawsuits against an employer) and adequate fulfilment of role responsibilities. Therefore, both to ensure productivity and quality of work and to protect himself against harm, the employer must be able to monitor aspects of the employer's work (Miller and Weckert, 2000).

Persson and Hansson (2003), in a discussion of arguments pro and con workplace privacy, point out that adequate performance by employees is not just a strong interest of employers, it is also something for which employers get paid wages and salaries and it is part of the contract that workers sign with their employees. As they emphasise, workers are accountable to their employers for their work. This entails a right to oversee that workers do their work, and do it properly. Many contracts even specifically sign over rights from workers to employees, often giving employers the explicit right to test or supervise the work performance of the employee. Persson and Hansson quite rightly separate this contractual obligation from a desire to make profits which is present in many organisations: clearly, non-profit organisations also have an interest in adequate work performance.

It can be concluded that the interests of employers and the obligations of employees present a strong case in favour of at least some monitoring of employees' work, arguably not only of work results, but also of the workplace itself (workplace surveillance). Persson and Hansson also identify two other arguments in favour of workplace surveillance. First, third parties, such as clients, sometimes also have interests or rights that may warrant workplace surveillance. For example, the management of a public transport corporation has a duty to reduce passenger risk as far as possible. This may require monitoring of drivers, including, for example, drug testing. Second, it can be argued that surveillance is sometimes in the interest of employees themselves. For example, medical tests and genetic screening can be used to protect the health of workers, and drug tests can help decrease drug use and thereby reduce the risk of workplace accidents. In conclusion, several good arguments can be made to restrict workplace privacy, based on rights and interests of employers, third parties such as clients, and employees themselves.

Arguments against Limitations on Workplace Privacy

The strongest and most straightforward argument for limitations on workplace privacy is undoubtedly the argument that employers have a strong interest, or even a right, to ensure good performance by their employees. I take this to be a matter of fact. The relevant question to be asked, however, is whether this right or interest of employers requires strong limitations on workplace privacy. If such limitations are not necessary to ensure good performance, then it is hard to see how such limitations on privacy could be justified. I have stated earlier that good performance involves quality and quantity of work output, doing no harm to the organisation, and adequate fulfilment of role responsibilities. It may be asked, then, whether the employer's interest in any of these three aspects of work performance requires strong workplace surveillance.

As for quality and quantity of work output, it would seem that close surveillance of workers often is not necessary to ensure such output. Clearly, there is no necessity to install surveillance cameras or monitor PC use and e-mail traffic if employers could also be asked to hand over their work output for inspection at the end of each day, week or month. The adequate fulfilment of role responsibilities by workers is sometimes more difficult to evaluate *post hoc*. But in most organisations managers have enough normal interaction with the employee, his or her fellow-workers and possibly clients to be able to know when an employer is not fulfilling role responsibilities. In most cases, therefore, close surveillance of the fulfilment of role responsibilities therefore seems unnecessary.

The prevention of harm to the organisation, which might result amongst others from carelessness, wastefulness, theft and embezzlement, clearly sometimes warrants workplace surveillance, as when there are clear indications that an employee is engaging in fraud or theft. In such cases, invasions of the employee's privacy, including searches and e-mail and telephone monitoring, may be justified. At issue, however, is whether the prevention of harm to the organisation justifies routine searches, routine e-mail and telephone monitoring, extensive camera surveillance, and so on. This would, indeed, be hard to justify as it would run counter to the way security is balanced against privacy and civil liberties in other sectors of society. For instance, police does not search your home or read your mail or tap your telephone conversations unless they have probable cause that you are engaging in illegal activity. The probable cause principle seems equally reasonable for workplace surveillance. If there is no probable cause that an employee is causing harm to the organisation, then there may be less privacy-intrusive means to protect the organisation against harm, like clear rules and procedures, company trainings aimed at improving safety, security and waste reduction, regular accounting checks and audits, tagging company property, and anonymised screenings of web and e-mail traffic. An exception may apply to heavily-regulated industries (*e.g.*, aviation, military and nuclear energy industries) and in organisations where employees have access to highly confidential records. In such organisations, a closer monitoring of employees may be required.

Background checks and tests that are performed as part of the hiring process seem to present a special type of workplace privacy issue. Here, it is not performance that is monitored, but the promise of good performance. The relevant question is: what types of personal information may an employer require in order to assess the prospects of good workplace performance? To answer this question, one must not just assess the privacy-sensitivity of certain types of information, but also their predictive value in assessments of employees. Moreover, issues of social justice and equality are also involved: is it reasonable for an employer to exclude employees because they have a genetic disposition to develop a certain medical condition or because they have a criminal record, and should employers therefore have access to such information? It would seem that privacy rights and considerations of equality and social justice impose serious limitations on the use of personal information in the hiring process.

I conclude that, so far, the burden of proof is on proponents of strong limitations on workplace privacy to demonstrate that such limitations are necessary to ensure good performance by employees and that alternative, less privacy-intrusive means to ensure good performance are not available. And it seems, so far, that such alternative means are often available. It may still be argued by proponents that contractual obligations or later agreements, voluntarily entered into by the employee, may void privacy rights. These contracts or agreements may for example specify that the employee is subject to certain types of surveillance, tests or searches. With such a contract, the employee obviously does not have a strong claim to resist such measures. But as Persson and Hansson rightly point out, such a contract does not void the moral obligation of the employer, which may sometimes also be a legal obligation, to choose those means for monitoring performance that are least privacy-intrusive. After all, as they point out, "The employee does not sell him/herself (that would be slavery) but his or her work" (63-64).

5. Conclusion: Privacy Rights in the Workplace

In my discussion of workplace privacy, I first presented an operationalised notion of privacy in section 2. Privacy was defined in terms of limited access to private affairs, after which three modes of access to private affairs were described (cognitive access, involving snooping or exposure, physical access, involving disturbances of private affairs, and informed control, involving the regulation of private affairs or wider aspects of someone's life). Next, five types of private affairs were distinguished, the human body, personal spaces and objects, bearers of personal information, individual conduct and social conduct, and it was claimed that these types correspond with different sets of privacy rights. In section 3, this operationalised notion of privacy was used to identify the main privacy issues in today's workplace. These are issues that range from genetic testing to video surveillance to e-mail monitoring.

In section 4, I then presented arguments for privacy rights in the workplace, followed by arguments pro and con restrictions on such rights. I concluded at the end of section 4 that while employers may have a strong interest in good work performance, it does not follow that strong limitations on workplace privacy are justified. Most arguments I presented for this position are not principled but practical ones: the fact is that strong limitations on workplace privacy are often not necessary to ensure good work performance. And if such limitations are not necessary, then it is hard to see how they could be justified. I have criticised one such justification that has been presented: that the limitations may be company policy and part of a contract that the employee has volun-

Philip Brey

tarily entered into. I have argued that organisations have a moral obligation, regardless of such contractual agreements, to ensure that privacy intrusions are not greater than necessary.

References

Alder, G., "Ethical Issues in Electronic Performance Monitoring: A Consideration of Deontological and Teleological Perspectives," *Journal of Business Ethics*, 17, 1998, 729-744.

Allen, A., "Coercing Privacy," *William and Mary Law Review*, 1999, 723-724.

Alterman, A., "'A Piece of Yourself': Ethical Issues in Biometric Identification," *Ethics and Information Technology* 5(3), 2003, 139-150.

Ball, K., "Situating Workplace Surveillance: Ethics and Computer-Based Performance Monitoring," *Ethics and Information Technology* 3(3), 2001, 209-221.

Bekkers, V., Koops, B. and Nouwts, S. (eds.), *Emerging Electronic Highways: New Challenges for Politics and Law*, The Hague, Kluwer Law International, 1996.

Brey, P., "Worker Autonomy and the Drama of Digital Networks in Organisations," *Journal of Business Ethics*, 22, 1999, 15-25.

Brown, W., "Ontological Security, Existential Anxiety and Workplace Privacy," *Journal of Business Ethics*, 23(1), 2000, 61-65.

Chadwick, R. Shickle, D., Ten Have, H. and Wiesing, U. (eds.), *The Ethics of Genetic Screening*, Dordrecht, Kluwer, 1999.

Cranford, M., "Drug Testing and the Right to Privacy: Arguing the Ethics of Workplace Drug Testing," *Journal of Business Ethics* 17, 1998, 1805-1815.

Dubbeld, L., "Observing Bodies. Camera Surveillance and the Significance of the Body," *Ethics and Information Technology*, 5(3), 2003, 151-162.

Fried, C., "Privacy," *The Yale Law Journal*, 77:3, 1986, 475-493.

Gilliom, J., *Surveillance, Privacy and the Law: Employee Drug Testing and the Politics of Social Control*, Michigan, University of Michigan Press, 1994.

Givens, B., "A Review of Current Privacy Issues," *Privacy Rights Clearinghouse*, March 2001.

Hes, R., Hooghiemstra, T. and Borking, J., *At Face Value: On Biometric Identification and Privacy*, The Hague, Registratiekamer, 1999.

Humber, J. and Almeder, R., *Privacy and Health Care*, Totowa, NJ, Humana Press, 2001.

Long, C. (ed.), *Genetic Testing and the Use of Information*, AEI Press, 1999.

McCahill, M. and Norris, C., "Watching the Workers. Crime, CCTV and the Workplace," in P. Davis, V. Jupp and P. Francis (eds.), *Invisible Crimes. Their Victims and Their Regulation*, London, MacMillan, 1999.

Miller, S. and Weckert, J., "Privacy, the Workplace and the Internet," *Journal of Business Ethics*, 28, 2000, 255-265.

Murphy, M. and Wilds, M., "X-Rated X-Ray Invades Privacy Rights," *Criminal Justice Policy Review*, 12(4), 2001, 333.

Nissenbaum, H., "Protecting Privacy in an Information Age: The Problem of Privacy in Public," *Law and Philosophy*, 17, 1998, 559-596.

Parent, W., "Privacy, Morality and the Law," *Philosophy and Public Affairs*, 12, 1983, 269-88.

Persson, A. and Hansson, S., "Privacy at Work – Ethical Criteria," *Journal of Business Ethics*, 42, 2003, 59-70.

Rosenberg, R., "The Workplace on the Verge of the 21st Century," *Journal of Business Ethics*, 22, 1999, 3-14.

Schoeman, F. (ed.), *Philosophical Dimensions of Privacy. An Anthology*, Cambridge, Cambridge University Press, 1984.

Simms, M., "Defining Privacy in Employee Health Screening Cases: Ethical Ramifications Concerning the Employee/Employer Relationship," *Journal of Business Ethics*, 13(5), 1994, 315-325.

van den Hoven, J., "Computer Ethics and Moral Methodology," *Metaphilosophy*, 28:3, 234-248, 1997.

Van der Ploeg, I., "Biometrics and Privacy. A Note on the Politics of Theorizing Technology," *Information, Communication, Society*, 6(1), 2003, 85-104.

Warren, S. and Brandeis, L., "The Right to Privacy," *Harvard Law Review*, 4, 1890, 193-220.

Westin, A., *Privacy and Freedom*, New York, Atheneum, 1967.

Wood, A., "Omniscient Organisations and Bodily Observations: Electronic Surveillance in the Workplace," *International Journal of Sociology and Social Policy*, 18(5), 1998, 136-174.

CHAPTER 6

Privacy, Discrimination, and Inequality in the Workplace

Sven Ove HANSSON

1. Introduction

One of the most widespread worries in connection with genetic test-ing is that it may give rise to discrimination, "genetic discrimination." It can, however, be questioned whether this term covers the important injustices that may arise in connection with genetic tests. The term "discrimination" is limited in scope, and there are many forms of unfair treatment of individuals that do not fit into that category. It is therefore important to put the discussion of genetic discrimination in a wider context. To what extent can medical testing, surveillance, and other privacy intrusions aggravate existing injustices or give rise to new ones? Which of these injustices take the form of discrimination, and what other forms of injustice need to be taken into account? How, if at all, is genetic information special in this connection?

It is the purpose of the present contribution to provide a preliminary answer to these questions, with special reference to the workplace context. Section 2 is devoted to the definition of discrimination, Sec-tion 3 to a characterisation of its wrongfulness, and Section 4 to deter-mining in what areas of social life non-discrimination can be enforced. Section 5 deals with how inequality and discrimination can result from the use of surveillance technologies in workplaces. In Section 6, the distinction between rational and irrational discrimination, that has previously been used in discussions on insurance, is applied to discrimi-nation in workplaces. Section 7 is devoted to a comparison of genetic and non-genetic information, from which it is concluded that regulations protecting health-related information should treat genetic and non-genetic information alike. A strategy for the combating workplace discrimination is outlined in Section 8 and in the concluding Section.

2. Defining Discrimination

"Discrimination" denotes that certain persons receive a worse treatment, or less of some advantage, than others, without sufficient justification to select them for such inferior treatment. However, discrimination does not refer to the *existence* of different treatments or to the fact that there are persons who do not receive advantages that others receive. Instead, it refers to the *selection* of persons for these different treatments. Someone can, for instance, complain that women are discriminated in the appointment of full professors, without having anything against the existence of full professorships or the privileges that are associated with these positions.

In contrast, "inequality" refers to the fact that some persons are in a worse position than others. Thus, inequality in work-life consists in the fact that some jobs are inferior to others. Hence, although discrimination and equality are often treated as the same issue, they are in fact distinct issues. There can in principle be inequality in a society without discrimination, and there can be discrimination in a society with a low degree of inequality.

In the cases that have attracted public attention, discrimination affects the members of certain groups, such as women, ethnic, religious, and sexual minorities. Adverse treatment can also affect a single person, but this is not normally called discrimination. (We have other words such as "harassment" to denote individual mistreatment.) As the term is used, "discrimination" refers to unfair treatment of the members of a group.

In all societies there are certain groups that are subject to discrimination, and the accumulated burden of discrimination is borne by the members of these groups. What makes discrimination an entrenched social evil is its repeated application to members of these groups. There may be single idiosyncratic acts of discrimination that are not part of a generalised social pattern. One employer avoids hiring people born on a Wednesday, for some superstitious reason. Another employer does not hire persons who come to the employment interview wearing jeans. A third does not employ vegetarians, *etc.* As long as these are isolated acts of discrimination they do not have the widespread social effects that the "classical" cases of discrimination have. However, if a superstition against persons born on Wednesdays started to proliferate, so that discrimination of these persons became a general social pattern, it would have to be taken as seriously as discrimination according to gender, ethnicity, religion, and sexual orientation.

120

One of the key issues in genetic discrimination is whether or not "genetic groups" can be identified, and subjected to repeated discriminatory action in the same way as the traditional discriminated groups. Unfortunately, historical examples show that this is the case. One such example concerns the recessive carriers of the sickle-cell gene in the Greek village *Orchemenos*. Since the gene was unusually common in this village, all inhabitants were offered testing. The purpose was to make it possible for carriers of the gene to avoid marrying other carriers. However, this strategy failed since testing led to stigmatisation of the carriers. Non-carriers chose to only marry other non-carriers, and carriers were left to marrying each other (Moore, 2000:107).[1] This example shows that the identification of a previously unidentified genetic group can lead to discrimination of the members of that group.

3. The Wrongfulness of Discrimination

The word "discrimination" is clearly negatively value-laden. More than that: it is essentially (or inescapably) value-laden. By this is meant that the negative value-ladenness is part of the word's core meaning. If you have said that a certain action is an instance of discrimination, then you do not have to add that it should not be accepted. Unacceptability is part and parcel of the meaning of discrimination (Radcliffe Richards, 1985).[2] Of course, there are many cases in which people receive different treatments for reasons that we consider acceptable, but such cases of differential treatment are not called discrimination. Hence, a person who is in favour of the connection between citizenship and suffrage would not call it discrimination that non-naturalised immigrants are voteless in parliamentary elections. On the other hand, the same person may very well call it discrimination if the healthcare offered to non-naturalised immigrants is inferior to that available to citizens.

But is discrimination wrongful *in itself*? It could be argued, with some plausibility, that only inequality is important, and that discrimination as such does not matter. From the viewpoint of the disadvantaged individual, the difference is not impressive between being disadvantaged

---

[1] Another example is the Ashkenazi Jews. This group has a long history of volunteering for genetic research, and therefore a disproportionate number of genetic alterations have been shown among them. This has given rise to a widespread though mistaken view that they are more prone than others to genetic disorders, and they have on occasions been discriminated for that reason (Dolgin, 2001).

[2] I refer here to the political sense of the word. There are other senses of "discrimination" that are not negatively value-laden. "A discriminating judge, a discriminating critic, or a discriminating collector, was a good thing to be" (Lucas, 1985).

due to discrimination and being disadvantaged due to "plain" inequality. How important is it that none of the groups to which I belong is treated (on average) worse than other groups, if I am myself treated worse than most other individuals? Some egalitarians have focused on the very existence of more and less advantageous positions, and considered the selection criteria for these positions to be relatively uninteresting side issues (Wilson, 1984).

But it is not as simple as that. At least two reasons can be given why inequality is a worse social evil when it is coupled to discrimination. First, there is considerable historical evidence that inequalities associated with discrimination are particularly entrenched. Discriminatory thought patterns become rooted in minds and in cultural traditions, and they are therefore much more difficult to eliminate than other sources of inequality. Each act of discrimination contributes to establishing or perpetuating a social pattern that will give rise to further wrongdoings. "All blacks have a chance of being discriminated against in future by a bigot whose racism is learned or reinforced by witnessing a discriminatory action" (Brooks, 1983). The second reason is that since discrimination expresses a negative appraisal of a group, an act of discrimination can be seen as a wrongdoing against all members of that group. Denying a person a job because of her ethnic background is an insult not only against that person; all persons with the same ethnic background may legitimately feel insulted by that action (Woodruff, 1976). These are strong reasons to give the elimination of discrimination a weight of its own, independently of its effects on inequality.

4. Discrimination and the Private Sphere

One of the most intriguing issues about discrimination is in what areas of human life non-discrimination should be enforced. It is easy to argue for such enforcement in public life. Public authorities should be fair in their dealings with citizens, from which it follows that they are required not to perform acts of discrimination. However, there are strong limitations to the enforcement of such principles in private life. Many acts that treat members of a discriminated group unfairly take place in the private sphere, in which we do not enforce the standards of fairness and equal treatment that are upheld in the public sphere. Our choices of friends and acquaintances are an example of this. A white family who never invites non-whites to visit their home may be prejudiced and bigoted, and could justifiably be criticised for their behaviour, but we would nevertheless consider them to be acting completely within their rights when choosing the company they wanted. "The pleasure of my company may, or may not, be one of the great goods, but it is for me to decide on whom to bestow it, however ardently you may yearn for it" (Lucas, 1985). This practice of non-interference is based on well-motivated principles of self-determination, but its effects are problematic since many small private actions can add up to a great social evil.

The social area in which we enforce non-discrimination is essentially the sphere of public life, in a relatively wide sense. This includes government organisations in their dealings with citizens, companies in their dealings with customers, sports organisations in relation to athletes, *etc.* The exact delimitation of this sphere of public life is far from simple, but for our present purpose it is sufficient to observe that workplaces belong to that sphere. Consider an employer who has racist leanings. As a consequence of this, he never invites non-white persons to visit his house, and he never hires non-white employees. He can defend the first of these habits by its being a private matter, but there is no such defence of the second habit. "The paradigm case of discrimination in individual action is generally taken to be an employer's appointment of a man or a white in preference to a woman or a black who is actually better qualified for the job which needs to be done" (Radcliffe Richards, 1985). Of course, discrimination in workplaces refers not only to hiring decisions but also to decisions affecting employees, such as decisions on promotions and salary.

Another way to express this is that the role of employing other persons is in a sense a "public office." A person who undertakes to be an employer thereby undertakes a social role in which she is required to fulfill certain criteria of fairness that are not required in private life.

5. Surveillance, Inequality, and Discrimination

Surveillance can be used to divide people into groups that are treated differently. Currently, surveillance of consumers is regularly used for that purpose. Internet activities and credit card records are utilised to classify consumers in categories that receive different offers and marketing messages from companies (Gandy, 1993). Insurance companies use medical information, including genetic information, as a basis for decisions that affect their costumers. The American insurance industry uses such information to reject applications for health insurance policies and to refuse payment for the treatment of illnesses (Alper and Beckwith, 1998). Commentators have feared that this practice can give rise to a "genetic underclass" of uninsurable persons (Anderlik and Rothstein, 2001). However, these problems are not universal but depend on the fragmentary nature of American health insurance.[3] Most European countries have more developed health insurance programmes. Since these programmes cover everyone, and premiums are the same for all persons on the same income level, there is no incentive for insurers to search for prognostic medical information about their customers.[4]

The potential for surveillance to give rise to social sorting and inequality applies to workplace monitoring as well.[5] In current practice, there are large differences in the degree to which employees are subjected to surveillance that may threaten their privacy. Surveillance does not take place in all workplaces. In most workplaces where it has been introduced, it does not include all workers.

In 1987, the Office of Technology Assessment (US Congress) performed a careful study of electronic workplace monitoring, in which the types of work-tasks most commonly subjected to monitoring were identified:

> Most of the electronic monitoring found by OTA and other researchers affects office workers with short-cycle 'production' jobs, that is, jobs where a limited number of standardized tasks are performed repeatedly to produce some information-based end-product. Most such jobs are considered clerical, for example data entry or insurance claims processing. However, monitoring can also be applied to professional jobs with a quantifiable output, for example computer programmers or insurance underwriters (Office of Technology Assessment, 1987:28).

The major criterion for electronic monitoring was "that the work be routine and require the repetitive performance of a small range of tasks." Therefore, monitored workers typically had tasks that "do not require a worker to have rare personal qualities, extensive professional training, or highly specialized skills" (Office of Technology Assessment, 1987:29).

However, OTA also noted that electronic surveillance was "increasingly being directed to higher level, more skilled technical, professional,

---

[3] Some commentators on the American health care system have claimed that the real issue is that of "a health insurance system that is built on sorting people into risk categories, and disadvantaging those most in need of health care" (Wolf, 1995).

[4] In Europe, since discrimination in health insurance is not an issue, discussions on genetic discrimination have focused on life insurance. Legislation and self-regulation have been instituted in several European countries in order to limit genetic discrimination in life insurance (Rosén, 1999).

[5] The distinction between surveillance of workers and surveillance of non-workers is not always sharp. Hence, camera surveillance of customers or the general public generally covers area in which some persons perform their work (Lyon, 2001:42).

and managerial positions" (Office of Technology Assessment, 1987:29). That tendency has continued, and at the same time the computerisation of non-office work has made it possible to monitor employees in many other types of work such as transportation, retailing, and industrial production. As was noted by Colin Bennett and Charles Raab (2003:40), it would today be misleading to believe "that those groups in society who have been economically and politically marginalized in the past... are more likely to be the subjects of higher levels of surveillance." The division between monitored and unmonitored work tasks does not coincide with traditional hierarchies on the labour market. Some of the heavily monitored employees are low-paid routine workers, such as call centre workers. Others are professionals with otherwise comparatively privileged positions, who just happen to have tasks that are easily amenable to electronic registration and measurement. There are similar conflicting tendencies in surveillance outside of workplaces. CCTV probably has its strongest negative effects on the otherwise underprivileged, whereas the surreptitious monitoring of consumer data is directed primarily at those who are believed to have money to spend.

From the viewpoint of preventing workplace discrimination it is important to consider whether or not workplace surveillance may be particularly burdensome for certain groups of employees. Physical surveillance of the body is in most societies particularly embarrassing for women, and it may also be problematic in certain subcultures and religious groups. However, there does not seem to be much motivation for intrusive monitoring of that nature.[6] Probably, a greater problem, and one that is much more difficult to deal with, is the difference between individuals in their reactions to surveillance. Some of us appear to be much more disturbed than others by being monitored. It is conceivable that these more "surveillance-sensitive" persons will have particular difficulties in some workplaces. However, they do not form an easily identifiable group. It is therefore probable that their situation will not be treated as an issue of discrimination but rather as individual cases of psychological problems.

---

[6] One exception is the use by the police (or anyone else) of concealed weapon detectors. These devices reveal images of all items concealed in or underneath a person's clothes from a distance of up to about 100 meters. Some of these detectors also reveal an image of the body's anatomical contours (Riley, 1997). The illegal activities of so-called "video voyeurs" who covertly videotape their victims in embarrassing situations give rise to similar concerns (Simon, 1997).

6. Rational and Irrational Discrimination

A useful analytical tool for the analysis of workplace discrimination can be appropriated from the discussion on genetic discrimination in insurance. The insurer's business is based on assigning different premiums to different individuals, corresponding to their estimated risk levels (Launis, 2000). From this point of view, a distinction can be made between rational and irrational discrimination in insurance. Rational discrimination is discrimination that accords with actuarial fairness, *i.e.* with the best possible estimates of risk levels (Anderlik and Rothstein, 2001). Irrational discrimination is discrimination that has no basis in actuarial calculations, and is therefore against the interests of the insurer. Obviously, this classification of a practice as rational or irrational does not imply a standpoint on its moral status.

The literature on genetic discrimination in insurance abounds with examples of irrational discrimination. Hence, patients with hereditary *hemochromatosis* have found themselves excluded from insurance although they complied with therapeutic phlebotomy and therefore had no increased risk of disease or death (Some relatives of patients with this diagnosis have avoided such discriminatory treatment by not having themselves tested but instead donating blood as often as phlebotomy is recommended for patients with the disease) (Barash, 2000). Afro-Americans who are carriers of the sickle-cell trait have been discriminated by life insurers, although their condition does not give rise to an increased risk of death (Bowman, 2000). (They have also been discriminated by employers; the US Air Force barred Afro-Americans with the sickle-cell trait from becoming pilots due to an erroneous belief that they were prone to illness at high altitudes (Dolgin, 2001).

The distinction between rational and irrational discrimination can be applied to workplaces as well. Just as insurers (in a non-universal insurance system) have a right to collect health information to determine the premium, employers have the right to select, among the persons applying for employment or promotion, those who have the best prognosis of successfully performing the job. We can call an act of discrimination by an employer rational if he has good reasons to believe that it is in his or her interest. Other forms of discrimination can be called irrational. Just as in the case of insurance, the rational/irrational distinction is descriptive, and should be distinguished from normative appraisals of the practices in question.

Many of the most discussed cases of discrimination in workplaces clearly belong to the irrational category, such as when an employer refrains from hiring the most qualified person because that person belongs to some minority group. Some forms of genetic discrimination fall under the same category, but there are also cases in which an employer's discriminatory use of genetic information should be categorised as rational discrimination.[7] Everything else being equal, hiring a person in good health is better for the employer than hiring a person with anticipated health problems.

Employers normally feel free to hire the person considered to be most fit for the job, and to make use of all information available to them in making that decision. Consider the following five examples of rational discrimination in a hiring decision.

The employer decides not to hire A because A will retire in three years, and a more durable solution is needed.

1) The employer decides not to hire B because B's health is bad.

2) The employer decides not to hire C because she is a young woman, and he has valid statistical evidence showing that young women often either leave the job after a few years, or demand a substantial reduction in working hours.

3) The employer decides not to hire D although her health is excellent at present, since non-genetic tests indicate that it may deteriorate within about three years.

4) The employer decides not to hire E although her health is excellent at present, since genetic tests indicate that it may deteriorate within about three years.

The first of these cases is probably the one that will give rise to least criticism. It takes some argument, however, to explain why the employer's behaviour in the other four cases should be criticised if we accept it in the first case. The third case is particularly illustrative. When we demand that an employer makes hiring decisions in a non-discriminatory way, we require that he hires the most qualified person even if that person belongs to a group known to have a higher statistical frequency of absenteeism, resignation, or other costly behaviours. Hence, we require that employers refrain not only from irrational discrimination but also from certain forms of rational discrimination. (Phrases such as "hire the most qualified person irrespective of gender and ethnic group" may give the opposite impression, unless one realises

---

[7] It has been hypothesised that it may in the future be possible to determine the probable sexual orientation of a person in a genetic test. The use of such tests in employment decisions would be a clear case of irrational discrimination. (The possibility of testing for sexual orientation has primarily been discussed in relation to prenatal testing. See Murphy, 1995 and Stein, 1998).

that it is not always in the employer's best interest to hire the most qualified person.) This confirms the observation, made in Section 4, that being an employer is in a sense a public office that involves obligations to sometimes set aside one's own self-interest when this is required in order to treat others fairly.

Cases 4 and 5 highlight the degree to which we consider genetic information to be more problematic than other types of medical information. Case 4 represents a practice that is more accepted than that of case 5. We tend to be more critical of the use of genetic than non-genetic information for employment selection, but do we have good reasons to treat the two cases differently?

7. Genetic Exceptionalism

It is not only in the workplace context that genetic information is taken to be more sensitive than non-genetic information. The same tendency is equally strong in the debate on discrimination in insurance. While it seems to be fairly accepted that an insurance company denies a person a life insurance who has a manifest illness with a bad prognosis, rejections based on genetic tests have been vehemently protested against. The view that genetic information requires more protection to ensure privacy than most other forms of medical information has been called genetic exceptionalism.

It is not entirely clear why genetic information is conceived so differently from the non-genetic information. Three major differences between genetic and non-genetic information have been invoked to defend genetic exceptionalism. First, genetic information is said to give more precise information about the likelihood of future disease than what is obtainable from non-genetic tests. Secondly, genetic tests give information not only about the tested individual but to some extent also about her relatives. Thirdly, genetic information is said to reveal fundamental and immutable characteristics of the individual (Alper and Beckwith, 1988).

As one example of the first argument (the predictive power of genetic tests), Roche and Annas claim that DNA-sequence data differs from other types of medical data in providing information not only about a patient's current health status but also about her future health risks, and that it is in this sense analogous to a coded "future diary" (Roche and Annas, 2001). This, however, is severely misleading. Although information about single-gene diseases may have a high predictive power, most health-related genetic information refers to diseases with a complex etiology involving several genes and several environmental factors. In such, more typical cases the predictive power of genetic tests is far from impressive. There are also several examples of non-genetic tests with a high degree of predictive power. Two practically important examples are blood pressure and occult fecal blood, that both have great value in detecting diseases (coronary disease respectively colon cancer) in their early stages before the patient is aware of it.

Although it is certainly true that family members can be affected by results from genetic tests, the same applies to non-genetic tests for infectious diseases (not least sexual partners in the case of sexually transmitted diseases). An interesting comparison has been made between Huntington's disease and HIV in this respect.

> *Inter alia*, Huntington's disease and HIV-positive status are analogous in that, at the time of diagnosis, victims of both diseases may have no symptoms and may remain healthy for a number of years; but even though the exact time of onset of both diseases is unascertainable, death of both victims within a given range of years is highly likely. Further, both Huntington's disease and HIV are transmitted to offspring at a relatively high rate (Gin, 1997).

Finally, genetic information is believed to reveal who the person "really is." The idea that we are defined by our genes has been called "genetic essentialism" (Alper and Beckwith, 1988). According to that view, genetic information is more intimately related to a person's true nature than other sorts of information about the person. As Launis has argued convincingly, this view is based on the highly controversial metaphysical presumption that there is such a thing as a person's core nature, or essential identity (Launis, 2000). Furthermore, the available empirical evidence shows that we are constituted by a combination of genetics and environment, not by genetics alone.

In conclusion, none of the common arguments for genetic exceptionalism seems to be tenable. There are many types of medical information that need to be handled with special care due its sensitivity with respect to privacy. Some but certainly not all of that sensitive information is genetic. The practical conclusions from this was excellently summarised by Green and Botkin:

> Tests that should be handled with caution include those that identify stigmatizing diseases, substantially affect family members, lack acceptable and effective treatments, and have results that are difficult for clinicians to interpret. Tests for Huntington disease, HIV, and inherited breast cancer, for example, raise all of these concerns... In effect, the justification for applying extra scrutiny to a test has little to do with the biological underpinnings of the disease or the method by which the information is obtained (Green and Botkin, 2003).

There are reasons to believe that future developments of non-genetic tests can make the current focus on genetic tests obsolete. There are already cases in which genetic information can be obtained indirectly through the identification of the protein produced by the gene, or through some other phenotypic indication of the activity of the gene. (As one example of this, a common cholesterol test can be used to diagnose hypercholesterolemia, a rare single gene disease characterised by extremely high cholesterol levels, Alper and Beckwith, 2000). With increased knowledge in proteomics, we can expect the number of non-genetic tests that correlate with genetic tests to increase dramatically. Furthermore, information about the expression of a gene can be more predictive than information about the presence of that gene. Therefore, non-genetic tests may very well be developed that have better predictive power than corresponding genetic tests. As one example of this, tests showing subclinical CNS effects typical of a certain psychiatric disorder may be more predictive than tests showing that the person belongs to a genetically defined group of persons with increased risk of that disease. The current focus on genetics may very well turn out to be counterproductive and to make us blind to serious problems of privacy connected with other types of biochemical information.[8]

8. Fighting Discrimination by Defending Privacy

The distinction between rational and irrational discrimination is highly relevant for the choice of policy instruments to curb discrimination. Since irrational discrimination is by definition against the perpetrator's own interest, it should in principle be preventable by making potential discriminators better informed of what is in their interest. On the other hand, rational discrimination cannot be defeated by appeal to informed self-interest. In the latter case, other enforcement methods will have to be considered.

Applying these principles to insurance, it should be clear that if insurance companies act rationally, then irrational genetic discrimination will be eliminated when they learn more about genetic disorders. A life-

---

[8] Several authors have warned that the current focus on genetic tests and genetic discrimination may lead us astray. Wolf (1995) refers to studies of ethnicity and gender showing that antidiscrimination analysis only gets part of the story. Instead of "genetic discrimination" she prefers to talk about "geneticism." Others have used the term "geneticisation" for similar reasons (Chadwich, 2000). It has been claimed that separate treatment of genetic information may increase the unmotivated stigma attached to genetic conditions and lend legitimacy to genetic reductionism and determinism (Rothstein and Anderlik, 2001).

insurance insurance company has nothing to gain from rejecting potential customers because of genetic traits that imply no increased morbidity. In contrast, we cannot expect rational discrimination to be eliminable by information alone. The success of a life insurance company depends on its ability to predict individual risk, using available information such as age, current health status including health-related test results, individual and family health history, occupation, alcohol and tobacco use, *etc.* (Anderlik and Rothstein, 2001). Asking the company to refrain from using all available information with a risk-predictive potential is tantamount to asking it to act against its own interest. Therefore, the only reliable way to prevent insurance companies from making discriminatory decisions based on a certain type of information is to deny them access to that type of information.

A similar argument applies to rational discrimination in workplaces. If it is in the employer's interest not to hire persons with a certain hidden condition or disposition, then the best way to prevent him from doing so is to block his access to such information. With respect to irrational discrimination, the situation is somewhat different in workplaces than in insurance. Whereas insurance decisions are made by specialised professionals, many employment decisions are made by persons with no special training for these decisions. There are also many more workplaces than insurance companies. In practice, it does not seem plausible that prejudices giving rise to discrimination will be eradicated among employers before they have been eradicated in the population at large. Therefore, in the case of workplaces, contrary to insurance companies, it seems necessary to apply the same strategy against rational as against irrational discrimination, namely to avoid as far as possible that employers have access to information that could be used as a basis for discrimination.

All this sums up to a very simple but also very important policy conclusion: *The most efficient barrier against discrimination based on (genetic or non-genetic) medical information is the barrier of privacy.* If we want employment and promotion decisions to be taken without regard to certain types of medical information about the individual employee, then the individual's right to privacy with respect to such medical information has to be upheld. This may require that it is made unlawful for employers to request such information about employees or employment candidates.

This strategy is much more easily implemented in Europe than in the US. The reason for the difference is that employers in the US often provide health care benefits not by paying premiums to an insurance company but instead by self-insurance. This means that the company itself acts as an insurer and directly covers the cost of medical services used by employees and their dependents. The self-insuring company has two overlapping roles, as an employer and as an insurer. In its capacity as an insurer it has all the rights of an insurer to obtain information from the insured person's (employee's) health records, including genetic information. Firewalls between these two functions in a company are not easily implemented (Gostin, 1997). The privacy problems associated with this arrangement will probably be aggravated in the near future by the inclusion in (electronic) health records of genetic information and other sensitive information for instance about neurobiochemistry. Such information will be needed for diagnosis and for individual selection of drugs and other therapies. In the American self-insurance system the potential for discriminatory misuse of health-related information is considerable. In Europe, the organisation of health insurance is more conducive to privacy protection, but measures may nevertheless be necessary to prevent employers from putting pressure on prospective employees to give them access to their medical records.

Finally, it should be noted that it is easy to get hold of enough tissue from a person to extract full genetic information about her. One obvious use such tissue samples is surreptitious paternity testing. Other uses are easy to think of. Workplaces are places where it is easy to get hold of samples of other persons' DNA. In order to protect individual privacy and prevent discrimination, the surreptitious acquisition and analysis of human biological material should be legally prohibited.

9. Conclusions

The following practical conclusions are offered as the outcome of the above deliberations:

- We need to consider not only discrimination but also other forms of injustice that surveillance and privacy intrusions in workplaces can give rise to. Discrimination and inequality are distinct issues that need separate attention.

- New inequalities arise in workplaces between the persons who are subjected to more surveillance, control, and privacy intrusions, and those who are not.

- "Surveillance-sensitive" persons who are more disturbed than others by being surveilled may have difficulties in heavily surveilled workplaces. Since these persons do not form an easily identified group it is probable that their situation will be treated as individual psychological problems rather than as an issue of discrimination.

132

- In work-life as well as in insurance, a distinction must be drawn between "rational" discrimination that is in the employer's economic interest and "irrational" discrimination that is not. Whereas discrimination of women and ethnic minorities is generally speaking irrational in this sense, discrimination based on valid medical prognosis may be rational, which makes it more difficult to eliminate.

- The employer's obligation not to discriminate employees or job applicants applies to "rational" as well as "irrational" discrimination.

- The most efficient (and possibly the only) way to prevent employers from making self-interested decisions based on medical information about employees is to deny them access to that information.

- The importance of protecting individuals from intrusions into their medical records will probably increase in the future due to the inclusion in health records of sensitive information such a full genetical sequences and the results of neurobiochemical tests.

- In view of how easy it is to get hold of a tissue from another person for genetic testing, legal restrictions should be introduced against surreptitious acquisition and analysis of human biological material.

- We can expect the development of non-genetic tests that have greater predictive power and are arguably even more sensitive in terms of privacy than genetic tests. Regulations that restrict access to sensitive health-related information should therefore make no difference between genetic and non-genetic information.

References

Alper, J.S. and Beckwith, J., "Distinguishing Genetic from Nongenetic Medical Tests: Some Implications for Antidiscrimination Legislation," *Science and Engineering Ethics*, 1988, 4:141-150.

Alper, J.S. and Beckwith, J., "On the Philosophical Analysis of Genetic Essentialism," *Science and Engineering Ethics*, 2000, 6:311-314.

Anderlik, M.R. and Rothstein, M.A., "Privacy and Confidentiality of Genetic Information: What Rules for the New Science," *Annual Review of Genomics and Human Genetics*, 2001, 2:301-433.

Barash, C.I., "Genetic Discrimination and Screening for Hemochromatosis: Then and Now," *Genetic Testing*, 2000, 4(2):213-218.

Bennett, C. and Raab, C., *The Governance of Privacy. Policy Instruments in a Global Perspective*, Aldershot, Ashgate, 2003.

Bowman, J.E., "Technical, Genetic, and Ethical Issues in Screening and Testing of African-Americans for Hemochromatosis," *Genetic Testing*, 2000, 4(2):207-212.

Brooks, D.H.M, "Why Discrimination Is Especially Wrong," *Journal of Value Inquiry*, 1983, 17:305-311.

Chadwich, R., "Ethical Issues in Psychiatric Care: Geneticisation and Community Care," *Acta Psychiatrica Scandinavica*, 2000, 101:35-39.

Dolgin, J.L., "Ideologies of Discrimination: Personhood and the 'Genetic Group'," *Studies in History and Philosophy of Science*, Part C: Studies in History and Philosophy of Biological and Biomedical Sciences, 2001, 32(4):705-721.

Gandy, O.H., *The Panoptic Sort. A Political Economy of Personal Information*, Boulder, Westview Press, 1993.

Gin, B.R., "Genetic Discrimination: Huntington's Disease and the Americans with Disabilities Act," *Columbia Law Review*, 1997, 97:1406-1434.

Gostin, L.O., "Personal Privacy in the Health Care System: Employer-Sponsored Insurance, Managed Care, and Integrated Delivery Systems," *Kennedy Institute of Ethics Journal*, 1997, 7:361-376.

Green, M.J. and Botkin, J.R., "'Genetic Exceptionalism' in Medicine: Clarifying the Differences between Genetic and Nongenetic Tests," *Annals of Internal Medicine*, 2003, 38:571-575.

Launis, V., "The Use of Genetic Test Information in Insurance: The Argument from Indistinguishability Reconsidered," *Science and Engineering Ethics*, 2000, 6:299-310.

Lucas, J.R., "Discrimination," *Aristotelian Society*, Supplement, 1985, 59:307-324.

Lyon, D., *Surveillance Society. Monitoring Everyday Life*, Buckingham, Open University Press, 2001.

Moore, A.D., "Owning Genetic Information and Gene Enhancement Techniques," *Bioethics*, 2000, 14:97-119.

Murphy, T.F., "Abortion and the Ethics of Genetic Sexual Orientation Research," *Cambridge Quarterly of Healthcare Ethics*, 1995, 4:340-350.

Office of Technology Assessment, "The Electronic Supervisor: New Technology, New Tensions," 1987, downloadable from http://www.wws.princeton.edu/~ota.

Radcliffe Richards, J., "Discrimination," *Aristotelian Society*, Supplement, 1985, 59:53-82.

Riley, L.B., "Concealed Weapon Detectors and the Fourth Amendment: The Constitutionality of Remote Sense-enhanced Searches," *UCLA Law Review*, 1997, 45:281-336.

Roche, P.A. and Annas, G.J., "Protecting Genetic Privacy," *Nature Reviews Genetics*, 2001, 2(5):392-396.

Rosén, E., "Genetic Information and Genetic Discrimination How Medical Records Vitiate Legal Protection," *Scandinavian Journal of Public Health*, 1999, 27:166-172.

Rothstein, M.A. and Anderlik, M.R., "What Is Genetic Discrimination, and When and How Can It Be Prevented?," *Genetics in Medicine*, 2001, 3:354-358.

Simon, R.I., "Video Voyeurs and the Covert Videotaping of Unsuspecting Victims: Psychological and Legal Consequences," *Journal of Forensic Sciences*, 1997, 42:884–889.

Stein, E., "Choosing the Sexual Orientation of Children," *Bioethics*, 1998, 12:1-24.

Wilson, W.J., "Race-Specific Policies and the Truly Disadvantaged," *Yale Law and Policy Review*, 1984, 2:272-290.

Wolf, S.M., "Beyond 'Genetic Discrimination': Toward the Broader Harm of Geneticism," *Journal of Law, Medicine and Ethics*, 1995, 23:345-353.

Woodruff, P., "What's Wrong with Discrimination?," *Analysis*, 1976, 36:158-160.

CHAPTER 7

Applying Ethical Criteria for Privacy

Anders J. PERSSON

1. Introduction

In workplace ethics, clear communication from theorists to practitioners is important if positive effects in the workplace are to be achieved. Technological developments have in many aspects improved work conditions, but at the same time new technologies have caused new problems for workers. Several practices infringe upon the privacy of workers. Some privacy invasions may be morally acceptable while others may not, and a crucial problem is how and on which grounds we are able to determine this. I will propose a set of criteria[1] for situations when intrusions into an employee's privacy are justified, and discuss three broad practices in relation to these: (1) Monitoring and surveillance – under which, if any, circumstances are, for example, monitoring of employees' use of telephones, electronic mail, computer terminals and the internet, morally acceptable? (2) Genetic testing – to examine workers for possible genetic predispositions may be a helpful tool of disease prevention, but is it morally justifiable to adopt such programs at the expense of privacy intrusions? (3) Drug testing – is it legitimate to override an employee's privacy by using such tests?

In relation to some scenarios on these themes, I will show that it is possible to handle such practical ethical problems systematically by way of the proposed guideline. The guideline offered can also be seen as an attempt to improve the communication from the theorist's side. Thus, managers will be able to make more consistent, more ethically accept-

---

[1] The criteria are to be found in Persson and Hansson, 2003. The presentation of these criteria, which tell us the ground for an ethical justification of privacy infringements, rests to a great extent on that article.

able decisions, when the scope of possible interpretations of infringements into workers privacy is restricted by a reasonable theoretical framework, which is defensible, practically workable, and can be easily grasped. A second aim is to show how certain practices, in relation to the criteria offered, emerge as dubious and how at least some of them can be replaced by less intrusive means of insuring for instance efficiency or safety on a workplace.

The first part will provide a discussion of what is meant by privacy and of what is special about workplaces in relation to privacy. Thereafter I propose that legitimate infringements of workplace privacy must be supported by justifications belonging to three categories. Each of these types of justification is discussed, and some important requirements for their validity are proposed. These criteria are then applied to three current practices, workplace monitoring, genetic testing and drug testing. In the concluding section the upshot of that application is summarised.

2. What Is Privacy?

An individual's privacy concerns the degree to which others may have information about her and sensory access to her. Privacy can refer not only to a person's body and mind but also to her possessions. However, not every type of information or sensory access to a person or his or her possessions can be the subject of *bona fide* claims of privacy. A person cannot, for example, legitimately claim that the colour of his or her outfit in a social setting it is a matter of privacy. This is the reason why a limited "sphere" around a person is often referred to in discussions of privacy. This notion is intended to capture the idea that the concept of privacy is only applicable within certain boundaries – partly, but only partly, of a spatial nature – that surround a person.

A crucial issue in the definition of privacy is the extent to which the boundaries of the sphere of privacy can be influenced by the individual's own wishes and preferences. Should a person always have preferential right of interpretation to decide what counts as an infringement of his or her privacy? Or should the individual's own wishes and preferences have no influence at all on what sensory or informational access to him or her is counted as an infringement of privacy? Both these views can easily be shown to have counter-intuitive consequences (Persson and Hansson, 2003). Therefore, a middle course between the two extreme views seems more reasonable. In what follows it will be assumed that the sphere of privacy consists of a *core* and a *discretionary part*. The core consists of such information or sensory access that is, in the relevant social setting, always counted as an intrusion into privacy. The discretionary part consists of those types of access that are considered legitimate for a person to wish to have control over. The contents of both parts of the sphere of privacy are of course determined by social traditions, and we can expect them to be different in different cultures.

The question whether "privacy" is a normative concept or not will not be discussed here. Instead it will be taken for granted that privacy is a normatively laden concept, but only to the level of *prima facie* moral principles. Although the notion of privacy can be used for purely descriptive purposes, it is then used to describe a system of social norms. A statement about privacy therefore is, or at least implies, a statement about norms.[2] However, it is not a statement about absolute or indefeasible normative status, but only one about *prima facie* normative status.[3] Like other *prima facie* moral statements, it can be overridden, but only when sufficiently strong justification can be given for the considerations that violate it.

An important conclusion to draw from this line of thought is that infringements of privacy always need a justification.

3. What Is Special about Workplaces in Relation to Privacy?

Since it seems to be a general idea that workplaces form a separate case that needs special treatment in respect of privacy infringements, something has to be said about what is so special about them.

The determining factor is arguably the employer-employee relationship as set forth in the contract of employment. The employee sells his or her work in accordance with such a contract. The contract of employment, understood in a wide sense, gives rise to *prima facie* obligations on the part of the contracting parties to fulfil both the conditions stated in the contract and the implicit, culturally determined, expectations of role performance in the work situation.

As stated before, the employee has a *prima facie* right to individual privacy. This means that legitimate intrusions into employees' privacy must have a justification, a justification based on what the employer can require of the employee according the contract of employment.

---

[2]   This means that privacy can be construed either as a normative concept or as a descriptive concept that is coextensive with normative ideas.

[3]   W. D. Ross famously developed the idea of *prima facie* duties. Such a duty is a moral obligation that is binding unless there is a stronger and overriding obligation. An actual duty, in contrast, is a remaining duty, all things considered. See Ross, 1930, chapter 2.

The employer's claim must, in other words, outweigh the employee's claim to privacy.

The employer's possibilities to fulfil this condition can be systematised into three categories: (1) the employers' own (business) interests justifies intrusions into workers' privacy, (2) the intrusion is justified by interests of the employee that the employer is required or at least entitled to protect, and (3) the intrusion is justified as a means to protect an interested third party's legitimate interests.

In summary, the criteria I propose are based on the assumption that legitimate infringements of workplace privacy must be supported by justifications belonging to one or more of these categories.

4. Ethical Criteria

From the contract of employment approach suggested here, it follows that the employer has the right to control that the work is properly done and that the employee fulfils his or her responsibilities. It seems uncontroversial that employers have some legitimate productivity expectations in virtue of such a contract. Nevertheless, even if employers' interests are supported by the contract of employment, arguably, intrusions into workers' privacy must also meet some other requirements, namely, those of minimal intrusiveness, efficiency, and limited severity.

If the employer can choose between different means to obtain the same level of control over the employees' work, it is a reasonable claim that only the least intrusive of the practicable means is legitimate. Naturally, it can be objected that this criterion offers a rather weak privacy protection, at least in practice, since it seems to leave unreasonably much room on the employers' side. The employer sets the agenda and has knowledge, power, control and the preferential right of interpretation concerning available means, one can object. However, the criterion should be understood in an objective meaning that makes it far more privacy protective than such objections suggest. For example, consider a case in which two means, A and B, are compared in terms of privacy intrusiveness. Suppose now that the employer comes to the conclusion that A is less intrusive than B, but more expensive to apply than the latter, and therefore chooses B instead of A. This choice can be described as if B was the least (practicable) intrusive means. In cases like this, however, the employer is not in general free to describe the situation as he or she wishes. This and the other criteria should be taken in a more objective or idealised meaning, which is analogous to the distinction between different kinds of reasons. The employer can be said to have a reason, R, to prefer B to A, based on his or her preference to save money. The proposition that R is a reason,[4] however, is a proposition that implies a much stronger claim on objectivity. If "least intrusive means" is understood in this latter meaning, then it is possible to reject, for instance, R, as a valid reason for implementing B instead of A. An ethical justification of an intrusion into an employees' privacy is possible only insofar as this criterion is fulfilled – *nota bene* – in this strict sense. A conceivable objection to this approach would be that it is indeed very hard to apply such claims on objectivity in practice. True, but that does not have effect on the reasonableness of the criterion as such. Besides that, it can also be argued that, at least in many cases, it would be quite clear which "the least intrusive means" is, objectively speaking.

Furthermore, for a privacy intrusive means to actually be in the employers' interest it must be an efficient means for that purpose. One might call the efficiency criterion in question, in a similar way as the foregoing one, and object to the employers' preferential right of interpretation. The reply is almost the same: "efficient means" should be interpreted from an objective point of view, which implies that we restrict the possible contents of the burden of proof rather strongly. Whether a certain means will become efficient, for a given purpose, is of course in many cases difficult to predict in practice. Nevertheless, objective evidence is needed in order to satisfy this criterion as well; the perspective should be that of an ideal observer. The proposed criteria should therefore be seen as ideals towards which the employer ought to strive.

Given that employees' interests should be respected, these interests have to be balanced against those of the employer. This means that even if a certain privacy invasive practice satisfies the criteria concerning efficiency and minimal intrusiveness, it still has to meet another condition in order to be ethically justifiable. The resulting intrusion into the employee's privacy should not outweigh the value of achieving its purpose. In other words, a certain privacy invasive means may well be both efficient for achieving its purpose and the least intrusive one compared to its alternatives, but despite that disqualified according to the criteria proposed here. The gain must also, reasonably, be balanced against the negative value of the intrusion in question. If the positive value, in terms of the employers' interests, is lower in comparison with

---

[4] This means, according to this terminology, that an invalid reason not really is a reason – objectively speaking. If one thinks that a certain reason *is* a reason and it turns out that it is invalid, then it neither is nor was a reason in this linguistic usage.

the negative value, in terms of invasions into employees' privacy, then the fourth criterion is not satisfied.

At this point one may wonder if this balancing of positive and negative values really is applicable at all in practice. As argued before, the criteria are proposed as ethical ones that tell us when an intrusion into an employees' privacy is justified from something like the point of view of an ideal observer. Naturally, in many cases it would in practice be presumptuous even to try to do such balancing. Nevertheless, my examples of practical cases will illustrate that it is both reasonable and possible to accomplish the bold estimates that are necessary for such balancing.

A justification with reference to the employee's own interests also has to meet the minimal intrusiveness- and efficiency-requirements. The essential issue to determine, according to the paternalistic relationship that the contract of employment implies, is whether the employer can be held responsible for work-related injuries or diseases. If that is the case, then the measures taken to protect the worker should actually be in his or her interest. To fire an employee when he or she could be relocated is an example of the opposite.

The last category, third party interests, refers to the interest of fellow workers, customers, neighbours to the workplace, and so on. Naturally, these groups can also have legitimate interests that can be balanced against the employees' privacy-related interests. As with the former category, the employer has to provide reasonable evidence that the intrusion in question actually has effects that meet the efficiency requirement. Obviously, the requirement of minimal intrusion is also applicable to this category of justificatory support for intrusions into workers' privacy. And, since both the employer's and the third party's interests should be considered, a balancing of these interests against each other seems to be reasonable for this category as well.

5. Some Comments on Ethical Criteria and Jurisdiction

Since the issues connected to the ethical approach presented here have also been discussed and elaborated at length by social scientists and legal theorists, it is important to take into account the privacy debate concerning law that has proceeded for over hundred years now.[5] However, since my approach to the workplace privacy issue is moral rather

---

[5] Warren and Brandeis' famous paper, "The Right to Privacy," is often referred to as a starting point for the legal discussion of "privacy."

than legal I will only make a few comments on how these approaches may relate to each other.

A common point of view among legal scholars is that the privacy of job applicants and employees ought to be protected. John DR Craig[6] has, among others, claimed that the law should provide a foundation of privacy protection for this category of people; the human right of privacy should be a part of this "floor of rights." He advances seven legal principles that should form the basis of a common approach of workplace privacy law in the countries discussed. The principles can be divided into two groups, one of which concerns the scope of application whereas the other concerns competing interests.[7] All these legal principles seem to be compatible with the proposed ethical criteria. The privacy protection available to employees depends, according to Craig, on "the legal source of the right to privacy."[8] Depending on the current legislation in certain countries some privacy rights can exist independently of the employment contract. Such rights can come into conflict with what is permissible according to a contract of employment. Other privacy rights can be limited by contractual agreement, and so on. Another aspect that, according to Craig, has reduced the impact of the legal right to privacy on employment law made the protection offered by the right [to privacy] highly circumstantial."[9] Craig's solution to this problem consists in the adoption of a principle according to which the (legal) right to privacy establishes a unified standard applicable to all employment relationships: "It should not be possible for employers and employees to contract out of the right, nor should candidates or employees be taken to consent implicitly or expressly to privacy invasions which would otherwise be unwarranted."[10]

The *moral source* of "the right to privacy" is plainly to acknowledge that privacy has a value, and therefore should be protected. From the very nature of privacy itself it seems to follow that a statement about privacy is, or at least implies, a statement about norms – not a statement about absolute or indefeasible normative status, but only one about *prima facie* normative status. If this is right, and if there is something in the idea that an individual's legitimate privacy expectations may differ

---

[6] In Privacy and Employment Law, there he considers the jurisdictions in Canada, France, the United Kingdom, and in the United States.

[7] See Craig, 1999, 143-70.

[8] *Ibid.*

[9] *Ibid.*, 156.

[10] *Ibid.*

in a working context compared to a non-working *ditto*, then the employer-employee relationship as set forth in the contract of employment seems to be the determining factor. A legitimate contract of employment gives rise to *prima facie* obligations on the part of the contracting parties to fulfil both the conditions stated in the contract and the implicit, culturally determined, expectations of role performance in the work situation. The contract of employment is thus, in my view, a proper basis for an ethical approach to the workplace privacy issue. From that basis one ought to consider the different interests involved, and limit intrusions into worker's privacy *via* reasonable conditions.

6. Guideline

So far, some preparatory work has been made for the ethical criteria that I am going to apply to six fictive cases. My intention is to show how theoretically reasonable criteria can serve as fruitful tools in practical application. The discussion aims at determining the moral status of possible infringements into workers' privacy related to the practices of workplace surveillance, genetic screening and drug testing. The following guideline[11] will be used as the theoretical basis for this.

An intrusion by an employer into an employee's privacy is justified if and only if it simultaneously satisfies all of the following four criteria:

1) The intrusion is undertaken with one of the following three purposes:

   a) to warrant that the employee performs the tasks and fulfils his/her responsibilities, owed to the employer, that are explicit or implicit in the contract of employment,

   b) to protect the employee's own interests in matters for which the employer is morally responsible, and to do this with means that are also in the employee's own interest, or

   c) to protect a third party's legitimate interests in matters for which the employer is morally responsible.

2) The intrusion is performed in a way that is an efficient means to achieve its purpose.

3) The intrusion is performed with the least intrusive means available to achieve its purpose.

---

[11] The criteria used are almost identical with the ones that are elaborated and argued for in "Privacy at Work – Ethical Criteria." See Persson and Hansson, 2003.

4) The resulting intrusion into the employee's privacy does not out-weigh the value of achieving its purpose.

7. Application of Criteria

7.1. Scenario – Workplace Surveillance[12]

Steven Walker is manager of an office, a unit of a large company. The balance sheet was returned recently, and it points at a substantial decrease for his unit. Steven as well as his superiors want to know the reasons for the disappointing result. He is also requested to present a plan for how the unit will be able to turn the red figures into black.

His analysis shows that the main source of the unit's financial problems is inefficiency. When thinking about this, Steven remembers an old school friend, Sheila Easton, whom he met on a reception a few days earlier. He was told that she is nowadays working for a software company that develops and markets tailor-made products for workplace supervision. A computerised controlling system may be a solution that also satisfies the company management, he comes to think. Steven decides to contact his old school friend.

After the meeting with Sheila he is aware of the huge amount of control that is available at a rather low cost.

Software programs can record keystrokes on computers and monitor screen images. *Via* such programs he is also able to have almost total control of individual PCs; the employees' mails and Internet activities will not be their private business any longer. Furthermore, telephone management systems can analyse the pattern of telephone use.

If Steven installs a software system that will allow him to monitor the work of each and every employee, it also allows him to bring the work of others on his computer screen so that he can watch individual work as it is being done. Steven can access copies of each employee's work at the end of each day and find out how much time each employee spent with the terminal off. He can review e-mail that the employee sent or received, and so on.

Steven considers the possibilities of using this tool and comes to think that he will show his superiors great ability to take action if he does so. On the other hand, putting all this information about the em-

---

[12] For more detailed examples of specific monitoring and surveillance technology for workplace use, see Rogerson and Prior, in Part III of this volume.

ployees together makes him feel uncomfortable. Should Steven use this software to monitor his staff?

If we start with the first criterion, *the intrusion should be undertaken with one of three purposes* specified above, it seems clear that it is satisfied in this case. Steven has worries about, and might have reason to believe, that not all of the employees fulfill their responsibilities. It could even be held that there are third party interests that would fulfill this criterion as well. The opposite would be the case if, for example, he decided to use the software tools just for curiosity or for the fun of it. Monitoring of employees without any reasons derived from the contract of employment could be labelled as harassment of workers.

Moving on to the question if the software programs are efficient means to achieve the purpose of increasing productivity, things become more difficult. (*The intrusion is performed in a way that is an efficient means to achieve its purpose.*) Is there reason to believe that the unit's efficiency will increase if monitoring is realised? At any rate, Steven has to carefully consider the consequences of using the different parts of the monitoring system. According to this criterion, parts that lack evidence for their efficiency to the intended purpose should be ruled out. Naturally, whether a specific monitoring tool in fact will be efficient or not is a difficult empirical issue. However, to fulfill this criterion, Steven has to upholster a decision to use such equipment with some evidence for its efficiency. At least for parts of the extensive monitoring it is highly unlikely that reasonable evidence can be presented. Therefore, the criterion is not satisfied in this case. The third criterion (*The intrusion is performed with the least intrusive means available to achieve its purpose*) is related to the second. It comes into play here if the former is satisfied, and it tells Steven that he also has to consider possible alternatives to the monitoring tools. If, for example, the productivity purpose could be achieved by means of education, information, reorganisation, changing of work routines, *etc.*, which would be less intrusive than the monitoring would be, the criterion is not fulfilled. Another suggestion, that would be less privacy intrusive, is plainly to measure work output instead.

If we accept the thesis that privacy has a value and that an employee has a *prima facie* moral right to individual privacy at work, it is also reasonable to accept that the value of this has to be balanced against the value gained from the employer's perspective. Suppose that Steven found out that all of the former criteria are satisfied. The last criterion (*The resulting intrusion into the employee's privacy does not outweigh the value of achieving its purpose*) then tells him to analyse anticipated (productivity) gains against the negative value of the intrusion into the privacy of his employees. If the gains are comparatively small in comparison with the losses, in terms of the negative value of privacy intrusions, this criterion is not satisfied. In other words, Steven must have strong evidence that surveillance would be a very successful tool in achieving its purpose, since there are, at least in a full-scale monitoring of the employees, reasons to believe that the resulting intrusions into workers' privacy would be very severe.

Needless to say, given that we adopt the presented criteria, it seems very hard to justify any extensive workplace surveillance. For example, monitoring of the e-mails that the worker has sent or received and his or her telephone behaviour can be counted as severely privacy intrusive. The employer has in most situations no rationale in thinking that such workplace monitoring is an efficient means, without less intrusive alternative, to achieve its (business) purpose. The prospective of an ethical justification of extensive workplace surveillance would, according to the proposed criteria, at least be very small. The outcome of this application of the ethical criteria is summarised in the table below.

Extensive Workplace Surveillance

1	Satisfied
2	Not satisfied
3	Not applicable
4	Not applicable
Conclusion	**Not justified**

Let us then make use of the distinction between surveillance and monitoring and modify the example a bit. The term monitoring can be applied to all automated collecting of information about work – regardless of purpose. "Surveillance," on the other hand, is narrower concept and refers to a relationship between some authority and those whose behaviour it wishes to control.

Following this distinction and the idea that not all monitoring is used for surveillance, we can alter the scenario. Steven can, for example, decide to install the software program, only aiming to collect information about employees' computer behaviour, without using it for surveillance purposes. Then, we will have the following table instead.

Workplace Monitoring not used for Surveillance of Work

1	Not satisfied
2	Not applicable
3	Not applicable
4	Not applicable
Conclusion	**Not justified**

7.2. Scenario – Genetic Testing

Wilma Harding works at the health and safety department of a major industrial chemical company. Her unit is engaged in elaborating a strategic plan aiming at strengthening workers' safety in general, and more precisely, to provide guard against work-related diseases caused by the dangerous chemicals handled by certain groups of workers.

One of the means proposed to accomplish that end is to use genetic tests. In genetic screening, workers are examined for possible genetic predispositions for example in sensitivity to chemically caused disease. In genetic monitoring, workers are tested for early genetic damage caused *e.g.* by exposure to chemicals in the workplace.

Wilma and the other members of the unit reflect upon a genetic screening program, which would be capable of identifying individuals who are susceptible to the chemicals used. This would be a powerful tool of disease prevention. Both job applicants and employees, who exhibit unfavourable genetic predispositions, could thereby be detected and protected from certain chemical exposures.

The members of the unit are well aware that there are several ethical and scientific difficulties conjoined with the practice in question. That intrusions into workers privacy might be a consequence of applying the program is one such difficulty. Wilma and her colleagues have some worries about that, and ask themselves: Under which, if any, circumstances would it be morally justified to apply such a genetic screening program? The purpose of adopting the screening program will certainly satisfy the first clause of criterion "1 b" – to protect the employee's own interests in matters for which the employer is morally responsible, and to do this with means that are also in the employee's own interest – to protect the employee's interests in terms of his or her health and safety seems to be sufficient for that. If the second clause, stating that the means must also be in the employee's own interest, will be satisfied depends on which policy Wilma's company will apply, if the screening tests identify persons who are judged to be susceptible to certain chemi-

148

cals at the exposure levels occurring in the plant. This point is stressed by, among others, Joseph Kupfer: "... relocating workers or modifying existing conditions so that they will be less hazardous takes time, effort, and money. It's plain cheaper to fire or not hire a worker who is at 'genetic risk'" (Kupfer, 1993:18). It is no easy matter to determine what measures by an employer are in the true interests of the employee. However, in relation to this case, the policy to be adopted must reasonably at the minimum imply that workers are not fired when they can be relocated. What is in a job applicant's own interests must, among other things, be due to what other job possibilities the job applicant has. In summary, the first clause of criterion "1 b" seems to be satisfied in this case. However, the second clause still calls for some sort of management policy in order to be satisfied.

As in the discussion of the former scenario, it is possible that a third party's legitimate interests might satisfy the first criterion. For example, an owner of a firm can be held morally and legally responsible for work-related diseases and injuries. Injuries on the plant can be costly for the owner in terms of both damages and bad publicity.

Even if the first criterion is satisfied, it still remains for Wilma and her colleagues to consider whether the genetic screening program is truly efficient and reliable. (*2. The intrusion is performed in a way that is an efficient means to achieve its purpose.*) The genetic screening practice, applied in a workplace context, can be questioned from different directions related to the efficiency-criterion. First, some commentators have worries about the reliability of the technique as such (Van Damme *et al.*, 1997). Second, even if the results from some genetic test are reliable, the results have to be interpreted through several instances before a decision can be made about an individual worker. Apparently, it is possible that this interpretation process, from the geneticist to the manager, could include several sources of error, and give rise to misunderstandings about how the results should be interpreted and managed in practice. Third, it could be questioned if the results emanating from this technology really are relevant for workplace safety. Susceptibility to a chemical substance and the risk a worker runs to contract a work-related disease are matters of degree. Even if the test has power enough to detect susceptible workers, it is not certain that any of them actually will develop the disease in question. They run a potential risk that in many cases would be hard to estimate with any precision. Of course, if all workers that run any risks were excluded from tasks involving exposure, then the genetic screening practice would, in one sense, be very efficient for its purpose. But since susceptibility is a matter of degree it would in another sense be inefficient, and also impractical, because all workers are susceptible to some degree.

Due to the working environment in the specific case, and the type of chemicals and the exposure risks they give rise to, genetic testing may well be an efficient means to purposes discussed in relation to the first criterion. However, Wilma and her friends may also have doubts on some other aspects of the efficiency of genetic screening.

Strongly connected to the discussion of the efficiency-criterion above, is the question if genetic screening is the least intrusive means to achieve the current purpose. (*3. The intrusion is performed with the least intrusive means available to achieve its purpose.*) If it were feasible (economically and practically *etc.*) to modify workplace conditions in a less privacy intrusive way, and achieve the same level of workplace safety, that would plainly be the alternative to choose according to the third criterion. This criterion seems very reasonable; if the employer has several alternatives, some of which are less intrusive than others – why not choose the less intrusive ones? In spite of this, it is quite demanding of the employee, since it requires that Wilma both makes an inventory of possible alternatives and weighs these against each other, in terms of intended ends and employees' privacy claims.

In a similar manner, according to the fourth criterion (The resulting intrusion into the employee's privacy does not outweigh the value of achieving its purpose), she has to weigh the value of applying the genetic screening program against the expected negative value of the privacy intrusions. There are also ethical problems that relate to family members of the tested employee. To even try to estimate such values is a peculiar thought, one might say. However, the information gathered from such tests can be handled in several ways, some less intrusive than others. If the information for instance were distributed to business colleagues, that would be more privacy intrusive than if the information were handled as strictly confidential medical information. Some categories of the employees, who are not exposed to any (hazardous) chemicals, such as messengers, office staff *etc.* can be requested to undergo genetic screening, or not. These options indicate at least that there are in fact some possibilities to compare negative values resulting from privacy intrusions. Theoretically at least, but I believe also in practice, comparison of the negative value of privacy intrusions with the positive value of achieving certain purposes, at the expense of individual privacy, can guide Wilma, and others in a similar situation, to ethically reflected and even justified decisions in this difficult matter.

Genetic Screening

1	Not satisfied
2	Not applicable
3	Not applicable
4	Not applicable
Conclusion	**Not justified**

Using the distinction between genetic screening and genetic monitoring the example can be modified. The purpose of genetic screening is to identify pre-existing genetic abnormalities, disorders or conditions in the genome of particular individuals. Certain decisions may then be made on the basis of the information obtained from such an analysis. Genetic monitoring on the other hand involves periodic examinations of an individual's genome to identify changes over time. The difference between genetic screening and monitoring has major ethical relevance. Although the information obtained through screening may benefit the employee by facilitating treatment, some forms have a purely exclusionary purpose. Genetic monitoring, in contrast, makes it possible to identify the environmental factors, which cause genetic disease, so that a vulnerable employee – and his or her employer – will be able to take steps to avoid these factors. Where the monitoring identifies an actual mutational activity in a subject, then there is much greater probability that continued exposure to mutagenic substances will lead to increased mutational activity.

Genetic monitoring may have a role to play in the promotion of health and safety. Tracking the health of employees exposed to substances with the potential to cause genetic harm may well serve as a protective tool. The early detection of mutational activity is made more likely by a monitoring programme that detects such alterations before they manifest themselves in physical harm. Protective genetic monitoring has not the same potential as genetic screening to be used to screen out employees who are disposed to genetic illness unrelated to employment. Certainly, genetic monitoring can only predict the likelihood of an employee or a job applicant becoming ill. Substantial privacy interests of the employee may be threatened by workplace genetic monitoring, depending on the uncertainty in the prediction, the timing and the nature of the illness. It may for this reason be problematic to meet criterion 2 as well as criterion 3. Nevertheless, the value of the information obtained from genetic monitoring would in many cases be comparable with the value of the information from testing of lead content in blood, and the

151

like. If methods and performance of the testing are carefully chosen, and high standards of confidentiality are satisfied, the use of genetic monitoring for protective purposes will satisfy the ethical criteria.

Genetic Monitoring

1	Satisfied
2	Satisfied
3	Satisfied
4	Satisfied
Conclusion	**Justified**

7.3. Scenario – Drug Testing

The management of a transportation company considers implementing a drug-testing programme. They are well aware that drug testing implies privacy intrusive social control. Nevertheless, there are strong reasons in favour of drug testing, in particular in business areas like theirs.

First, strong third party interests, first and foremost the safety of passengers and fellow road users, can be boosted. Second, a drug testing policy can be motivated by the employer's responsibility for the employees' own health and safety. A purpose relevant to the safety of both third parties and the employee her- or himself is also that drug testing may deter employees from using drugs, and from becoming safety risks. Third, business interests can also motivate such a policy since drug abuse among the employees would in many respects be bad for the company. "Overall, a strong drug testing policy shows to both customers and employees that the company takes the drug issue seriously," says one of the managers. Most of the others in the management group agreed. After some discussions four policy options seemed to be available:

(a)   Testing of all employees or (b) employees in certain categories.

(a)   Testing without cause (no basis for believing that the subject is a drug user is required) or (b) testing with cause (such a basis is required).

(a)   Universal (all employees in the selected groups are tested) or (b) random testing.

(a)   Non-scheduled testing (without notification in advance) or (b) testing after advance notice.

Assume that the "(a)"-alternatives above was chosen. The testing policy will then be that all employees, universally, will become subjects to surprise testing without any claim on reasonable suspicion for drug use. Can such a policy meet the ethical criteria suggested?

The first criterion, telling that the intrusion should be undertaken with one of the three purposes mentioned above, is certainly satisfied in this case. Third parties such as passengers seem to have legitimate expectations on a certain level of safety, which reasonably involves that drivers and pilots not are under influence of liquor or other drugs while performing their job tasks. The purpose of protecting the employee's own interests is also likely to be satisfied in cases like this, both for plain safety reasons and for other kinds of reasons related to "the employee's own good."

Whether the *intrusion is performed in a way that is an efficient means to achieve its purpose* can, however, be called in question. First, the accuracy of drug tests has been subject of criticism from several commentators (Manfield, 1997; Feldthusen, 1988). False positives may not be problem for achieving the purpose of protecting a third party's interest,[13] but they certainly are so concerning the purpose of protecting the employee's own interest. If the drug test implies a potential risk for the employee to be weeded out without grounds as a drug user then it cannot be in the employee's own interests to be tested. Whether the drug test policy in question is an efficient means to deter employees from drug use is a difficult empirical question to answer. We can expect the degree of deterrence efficiency to depend on the form of testing adopted. The strong testing policy ("the a-alternatives) is probably the best candidate for this, and may therefore satisfy the efficiency criterion.

The intrusion is performed with the least intrusive means available to achieve its purpose. Is this criterion satisfied as well? The form of policy seems to be important for the answer to this question. Universal testing of all employees without cause includes testing of employees who constitute no particular risk to third party interests. The risk that an intoxicated ticket clerk causes damage to fellow employees and passengers is probably very low. On the other hand, the risk associated with a bus driver or airplane pilot who is under the influence of drugs or alcohol may be very great, when one considers the lives that could be lost in a drug-related accident. In order to prevent such accidents the drug test

---

[13] Certainly, if the reliability of a certain drug test is very bad, so bad that it become generally known that several false positives are picked out, then it will be problematic to achieve this purpose.

policy in question may well be both effective and the least intrusive means available – for "high risk-categories," but not for "low risk-categories." Therefore, universal testing of all employees cannot be considered as the least intrusive means in this case. For example, testing of employees in certain categories is an available means that would be less intrusive.

Universal Drug Testing of All Employees

1	Satisfied
2	Satisfied
3	Not satisfied
4	Not applicable
Conclusion	**Not justified**

Let us see then if the problem of satisfying the least intrusive means-criterion may be solved by a modification the drug testing policy.

Suppose that the management is able to distinguish between "high-risk" and "low-risk" categories of employees. Then a restricted policy is possible (in compliance with the "b"-alternatives above): (1) Testing only of employees in certain (high-risk) categories, (2) the employer is required to have a reasonable basis for believing that the subject is a drug user, (3) the tests are randomly performed with a cause, and (4) tests are notified in advance.

A more restricted policy like this will also satisfy the first criterion. The second criterion, if *the intrusion is performed in a way that is an efficient means to achieve its purpose*, is, however, not as easily determined. A possible consequence of the more restricted policy is that it would be less deterrent than the one discussed above, and due to that less efficient to achieve its purpose. The conditions of the restricted policy make it easier to avoid undergoing a drug test as well as passing a test, form the perspective of the employee. This policy can therefore, in regard of prevention, be accused of lacking efficiency for its purpose. Nevertheless, it can be said to be an efficient means to identify drug users on a workplace. Presumably, the criterion will be satisfied with regard to the all the purposes of the first criterion.

Whether the present drug test policy will solve the problem of satisfying "the least intrusive means-criterion" depends on the reasonable alternatives open to the employer. The employer should be able to show that there is no less intrusive method to achieve the purpose of protecting the employee's own interests as well as third party interests on this matter. Other forms of control, that are less privacy intrusive, and information programs have to be ruled out as not as good for achieving the purpose of protection. Only if that is the case, the criterion will be satisfied.

Last, given that the employer manages to show that the means chosen are the least intrusive one, the criterion that *the resulting intrusion into the employee's privacy does not outweigh the value of achieving its purpose*, comes into play. The manner in which drug testing is carried out and how the information from such testing is handled, are relevant for this balancing. The severity of the privacy intrusion has to be compared with the prospect and the value of achieving the purpose of the drug test. If, and only if, it is reasonable to accomplish consequences of the policy that promote the employee's own interests and/or third party interests, to a degree that outweighs the loss of privacy, the last criterion will be satisfied. At least if the other criteria are carefully considered and complied with, there seem to be good prospects of doing that. This applies in particular when, as in this scenario, the policy adopted is restricted to the special categories of employees. The lives that could be lost if a drug-related accident were to occur can surely motivate privacy infringements to some degree on, for example, bus drivers and airplane pilots on behalf of third party interests.

**Restricted Drug Testing for Employees
with Safety-sensitive Tasks**

1	Satisfied
2	Satisfied
3	Satisfied
4	Satisfied
Conclusion	**Justified**

8. Conclusion

The fictive cases presented above are of course very schematically described and lack a lot of technical and practical information that would be relevant in real cases for an ethical justification of privacy intrusions on workplaces. Nevertheless, the discussion of these scenarios, in relation to the proposed set of criteria, indicates that some current practices are dubious, and also that some of them can be replaced by less intrusive means of achieving efficiency or safety on a workplace.

In conclusion, if one finds the proposed ethical criteria reasonable, then one also has reason to believe that the objectives for which employers' use some of the more intrusive modern technologies can and should be met with far less privacy-intrusive means. The same seems to be true about the way that such tools are handled in practice. The proposed guideline can be used by the employer for determining whether or not a certain privacy invasion is morally acceptable.

References

Craig, J.D.R., *Privacy and Employment Law*, Oxford, Hart Publishing, 1999.

Feldthusen, B., "Urinalysis Drug Testing: Just Say No," 5 *Canadian Human Rights Year Book* 81, 1988.

Kupfer, J. H., "The Ethics of Genetic Screening in the Workplace," *Business Ethics Quarterly* 3(1), 1993, 17-25.

Manfield, K., "Imposing Liability on Drug Testing Laboratories for 'False Positives': Getting around Privacy," *The University of Chicago Law Review*, 64(1), 1997, 287-315.

Persson, A. J. and Hansson, S.O., "Privacy at Work – Ethical Criteria," *Journal of Business Ethics* 42, 2003, 59-70.

Ross, W. D., *The Right and the Good*, Oxford, The Clarendon Press, 1930.

Van Damme, K. *et al.*, "Ethical Issues in Genetic Screening and Genetic Monitoring of Employees," *Annals of the New York Academy of Sciences* 837, 1997, 554-565.

Warren and Brandeis, "The Right to Privacy," *Harvard Law Review* 193, 1890.

CHAPTER 8

The Dimensions of Privacy

Elin PALM

1. Introduction

The development within surveillance technology leaves fewer and fewer private spaces where individuals may remain anonymous and free from intrusion. Surveillance can be operated by *e.g.* computers, positioning systems, biometric identification, and biomedical tests and can cover most aspects and areas of work. In the workplace, individual employees' activities can be displayed, documented and analysed in detail. Novel forms of surveillance and 'surveillance capable technology' (see chapter 3) necessitate renewed analysis and discussion of privacy and privacy protection. A large part of the privacy intrusions caused by workplace monitoring could probably be avoided with a better understanding of the elements that contribute to intrusions.

Two common ways of addressing privacy issues posed by workplace monitoring are privacy compliance audits and Privacy Impact Assessments (PIA). Whereas a privacy compliance audit presumes existing legislation with which a proposal or project must comply, a PIA adopts a broader perspective considering the impacts of a certain practice that is independent of prevailing legislation.[1] But even though certain "privacy critical points" worthy of assessment have been identified, little has been said of why technologies/practices are privacy intrusive and how the type of information obtained corresponds with perceived privacy intrusiveness. Important questions remain: at what stage does workplace monitoring become invasive and what characterises privacy infringements?

In this paper, a dimensional analysis is proposed as a means to identify actually or potentially privacy invasive monitoring practices. A

---

[1]   See http://www.anu.edu.au/people/Roger.Clarke/DV/PIA.html.

central aim is to analyse the ways in which different types of monitoring intrude upon employees' privacy in order to guide the evaluation of workplace monitoring. The dimensional analysis can contribute to better solutions to the problems that workplace monitoring intends to solve. Even though negative implications cannot be avoided altogether, by means of the proposed analysis, negative implications can be alleviated and minimally intrusive means of monitoring identified.

2. Privacy

Although the concept of privacy is frequently used and although it generates an intuitive understanding, a precise definition is difficult to reach. On a theoretical level, *i.e.* in legal and philosophical discussions on privacy, little unity is to be found. Two significant approaches can be extracted however; either privacy can be understood in terms of separation or in terms of control.[2]

The separatist view can be exemplified with how privacy has been described in terms of a right to be left alone and how it has been interpreted as seclusion. In the latter case, a person experiences privacy when she has withdrawn to a place where she is neither looked at nor listened to (Thomson, 1975). Often, privacy is described in terms of a private sphere where the individual ought to be left alone (*e.g.* Westin, 1967:7), that is, where she is justified in expecting freedom from intrusions of various kinds.

The control-oriented view emphasises the importance of individuals' ability to control information about themselves and others' access to certain aspects of them, *e.g.* control over a zone in which the individual can be free from certain types of intrusion (Scanlon, 1975:316). One reason for emphasising the importance of control over personal information is the understanding of privacy as an important instrument for social living *i.e.* that there is a close connection between our ability to control others' access to information about us and our ability to create and maintain different sorts of relationships (Rachels, 1975:326). It is not others' lack of information about us that implies privacy, "[r]ather; it is the control we have over information about ourselves" (Fried, 1984:209).

The separatist view seems problematic in the sense that it fails to distinguish privacy from other important values tied to it. Where privacy is

---

[2]   It should perhaps be noted that the differences between these lines of reasoning are more a question of emphasis than of fundamentally different views.

understood as a right to be left alone, privacy is confused with liberty and where privacy is interpreted as seclusion, with solitude (Tavani, 1999:266). More importantly however, in many cases we do not want to be left alone or secluded, but still we want to be able to claim privacy.

An adequate concept of privacy should take into account our need to be private in public. To the contrary, privacy is most often discussed in terms of a sharp distinction between the public and the private. When emphasising a basic human need to be able to withdraw from public life to a private sphere, it has almost been taken for granted that privacy in public is something contradictory. "For the majority of theorists, it follows seamlessly that the concept and the value of privacy corresponds with, or applies to, the sphere of the private alone" (Nissenbaum, 1998:568). This dichotomy is too sharp, excluding the possibility of reasonable expectations on privacy in public and *semi*-public areas like the workplace. Such expectations are often discarded as practically impossible. A dichotomy between individual and society, or between private and public fails to recognise that people operate in a range of contexts where they are more or less private (Regan, 1998:32). Even though Warren and Brandeis, in an early discussion on privacy, sought to defend celebrities' "right to be left alone" *i.e.* to remain reasonably private despite their status as public persons (Warren and Brandeis, 1890), attempts to secure privacy in public have been sparse thereafter.[3] To the extent privacy in public is discussed, it is primarily confined to specific institutionalised relations, *e.g.* between lawyer and client, physician and patient, teacher and student *etc.* According to such an understanding, privacy is violated when someone acquires information about me that she is not entitled to, by virtue of her relationship to me.

The control-oriented view is also saddled with certain problems. Control in the sense of being able to deny others' requested privacy sensitive information about oneself, or otherwise to take action to prevent others' from obtaining private information they obviously seek to obtain does not necessarily eliminate the intrusiveness. Having to take action in a way that one preferably would not have to do but that is necessary in order to feel comfortable can in itself be an infringement of privacy.

A central aspect of privacy protection following the control-oriented view is that of being able to adopt an appropriate behaviour (*e.g.* Rachels, 1975:331). However, in the long run, adjustment is most likely

---

[3]   For interesting discussions on privacy in public, see abovementioned articles by H. Nissenbaum and P. M. Regan.

an unsuccessful way of dealing with others' access to information about oneself. In an aspiration to gain acceptance and liking, individuals may alter their behaviour to an extent they would prefer not to do. In a situation where employees are subjected to camera surveillance, they may try to second-guess the "panopticist" and adopt an allegedly appropriate behaviour. Of importance here is whether the employees can respect the view of the supervisor or not. It is decisive if individuals adjust to a norm that they can accept (Williams, 1994:82). Over time this adaptation may invoke a feeling of having given up something valuable of oneself when having adjusted to a norm assumed to prevail and maybe not even embraced.

The tendency to let the individual govern her privacy is clad with several problems. The task of defining the borders of one's sphere of privacy can be left to the individual. Then, the individual delineates the borders of her private sphere and her experience of those borders being trespassed is what *de facto* constitutes a privacy intrusion. According to such an understanding individuals can choose to make do with a minimal sphere of privacy and waive or neglect reasonable privacy claims. In consequence, docu-soap participants who allow TV-watchers total insight in their doings over a certain period of time still maintain their privacy. And in a similar vein, job applicants could be free to trade off as much of their reasonable privacy claims as they choose to when signing employment contracts.

This understanding of privacy seems to underestimate the force of social expectations. To a large extent, privacy is culturally and customary defined. Even if I exercise control in the sense that I choose to openly display my health-register, it seems difficult to hold that I have my privacy intact since this information is generally considered to be private affairs. Hence, I would argue that the abovementioned persons have lost their privacy.

Furthermore, the individual's consent plays an important role in the control-oriented approach. However, the tendency to assert weight to consent without taking into account the situation in which it is given is problematic. Privacy is insufficiently protected by a system in which privacy is completely dependent on an individual's consent or denial to reveal information about herself. By accepting to undertake a drug test, a prospective employee has not by necessity given her consent to the practice. Neither, does her acceptance to undertake the test in question eliminate the privacy intrusive element of the practice. Out of self-interest, a prospective employee may consent to certain tests that she would otherwise have refused.

Even though I will emphasise control over and ability to limit or restrict others' access to information about oneself (both immediate sensory information and collected data) as an important aspect of privacy, individual control is insufficient to protect privacy. Rather than letting individuals define the borders of privacy intrusions, it will be held forth that there is a certain limit beyond which individuals should neither be expected nor accept to waive their reasonable privacy claims. As proposed by Anders Persson and Sven Ove Hansson, a certain core of information ought to remain with the person irrespectively of what claims she makes (Persson and Hansson, 2003:62-63). In the workplace context, certain information should not be required from the employee. Most people react negatively to pre-employment drug tests and pregnancy tests (Marx, 1998:173). The negative reactions to such practices should be considered morally relevant, especially since employees have difficulties refusing to give up personal information.

To sum up, assuming that privacy is a morally relevant interest that need (better) protection, my primary aim with regards to privacy is to amplify the relevance of taking privacy expectations in public and in *semi*-public areas seriously and to emphasise a need for respect for non-articulated but reasonable privacy claims.

3. The Features of Privacy Intrusions

Even though employers need a certain degree of monitoring of workplace activities as well as a certain amount of data collection about employees in order to ensure a safe and productive workplace, the moral costs in terms of privacy intrusiveness can be high. The relations between employer and employee may be strained, trust negatively affected, spontaneous actions and initiatives stifled *etc.* as a result of inconsiderate ways of seeking the information needed. Certainly, employers are entitled to certain information about their employees – but what kind of information and what sensory access, and under what conditions? In order to clarify some important aspects of how workplace surveillance may affect individuals, I will distinguish between various features that characterise a privacy intrusion. A dimensional analysis will be introduced in order to avoid unnecessary privacy intrusions and to identify the least intrusive means of monitoring. Its major dimensions are based on seven questions that ought to be addressed when a new surveillance method or device is to be implemented:

Type: What type of information is made accessible?

Purpose: Why is the information collected?

Excess: Is surplus information obtained?

Storage: How, if at all, is information stored?

Access: Who has access to information?

Awareness: Is the person under surveillance informed?

Influence: To what extent can individuals influence surveillance?

The above-mentioned questions are motivated by experiences from problematic applications of surveillance capable technology and the grave moral costs where a monitoring device has been implemented and used in an improper way. These aspects have proven to be crucial with regards to privacy intrusions in the past and need to be recognised at an early stage of implementation. The dimensions listed are intended to cover the critical issues that monitoring tends to give rise to (since coverage has been given priority, some of the dimensions may overlap). These issues are all ethically relevant and can be motivated as important irrespective of what philosophical starting-point one takes. The dimensions can be used both to guide the implementation of surveillance capable technology and to assess established monitoring practice.

Type

Whereas earlier surveillance technology foremost served to monitor groups of people, modern technology enables detailed maps and descriptions of individuals' behaviour. In the case of workplace monitoring, an individual employee's work performance can be measured by means of "Bigbrotherware" *i.e.* software programs recording keystrokes, monitoring exact screen images and time spent on certain websites. Such programs give managers almost complete information about individual PCs and individual work patterns. Furthermore, location based technologies enable employers to identify an employee's location and trace her movements. Smart cards equipped with Radio Frequency ID (RF ID) are frequently used on workplaces and are increasingly often combined with information that enables biometric authentication in order to facilitate employees' access to computers and locked areas. At the same time, such cards enable real time tracking of employees' physical movements within the building. Geographic Information System (GIS) technologies can locate and trace workers regardless of where they are *e.g.* by means of company cell-phones. Hence, employees need not even be present at a traditional workstation in order to be subjected to monitoring.

Within medical technology, tests have been developed that reveal predispositions to certain diseases. Biological monitoring of work-related exposures by means of urine or blood samples is part of occupational health practices in work with some hazardous chemicals *e.g.*

organic solvents or metal compounds. Health surveillance can be used to reduce hazards on the workplace but information about an employee's genetic disposition can also be used to estimate her future work capacity and to exclude job applicants or deny promotion on the basis of predicted future health. Furthermore, employees, present or prospective, may be subjected to AIDS tests, pregnancy tests and drug tests.

There seems to be certain information that most people would agree that the individual is justified in keeping to herself (in case no important right is violated thereby). Sexual orientation, religious beliefs or affiliations, political opinion or association membership, genetic information and health information are examples thereof. Since these data can, in certain contexts, be socially stigmatising if openly displayed, individuals should not be required to state such information. Julie. C. Inness has argued that information that concerns private matters that individuals care for is to be regarded as privacy sensitive and the core of privacy has been identified as intimacy (Inness, 1992:7). In the workplace context however, information that not necessarily is to be characterised as intimate can be privacy sensitive, due to the imbalanced (power/dependency) relation between employer and employee. As noted by James Rachels, the importance of control does not exclusively concern information that is too intimate to share, or embarrassing to exposure (Rachels, 1975:325). Certainly, information that is considered privacy sensitive in society at large is most likely sensitive in the work place context as well, *e.g.* nudity. The collection of urine samples for drug testing is criticised for being unduly privacy invasive since these tests are carried out under supervision in order to prevent tampering (Carson, 1995:3-4). In addition, certain types of information become privacy sensitive in the workplace *e.g.* due to the ability to, continuously, collect and store information about individuals. By using the abovementioned monitoring practices as examples, four subcategories of information that is likely to be privacy sensitive within the workplace can be extracted.

A first subcategory of potentially privacy sensitive information is *bodily information*, including both the genetic constitution of an individual and her physical features. The results of psychological tests, IQ tests and genetic tests revealing information about ones capabilities or identity are also privacy sensitive. In particular, genetic tests are thought of as revealing something fundamental about an individual's identity. Biological information laid bare by genetic screening is seen as inherently personal. The information is considered especially sensitive since an individual's genetic dispositions can be used to control her access to job opportunities even though she cannot alter or improve her genetic make-up (Rosenberg, 2000:89). Connected with information about our

163

genetic disposition (revealed by predictive genetic testing) is also the question of a right not to know about one's future (Häyry and Tukala, 2001). Some people prefer to remain ignorant with regards to what "their future looks like" and they may not want others to know about this either.

A second information type to be considered is *location and movements*. Concomitant with more flexible work forms, such as distance work, surveillance technologies capable of identifying workers' location are taken in use. Location-based technologies enable both identification of a worker's geographical location and tracing of her movements within an office building or by a company car. The technology can measure the amount of time a service worker spends in travelling between scheduled visits. It can be assessed if she goes straight from one visit to another, if the shortest way is chosen *etc.* Information about one's location at a certain time may be perceived as privacy sensitive information. Having one's movements mapped and analysed is generally perceived as even more privacy sensitive.

A third subcategory is information concerning *habits and behaviour*. Modern surveillance-capable technologies are to a large extent automated, allowing for continuous recording of all activity within a certain area – information that would otherwise be inaccessible (Tunick, 2000:268). *E.g.* the Hygiene Guard® provides employers with information about employees' hygiene behaviour.[4] The employee's identity badge activates a sensor when entering the toilet and another when leaving. In case the employee has not turned on the faucet and used the soap dispenser before leaving, this will be registered and may lead to acts of reprisals.

Video monitoring provides complex information about frequent bypassers. As long as the occasions when one passes a surveillance camera remain isolated events, monitoring is not seen as very intrusive. However, within a confined area such as the workplace, where people find difficulties to avoid the "panopticist's gaze," continuous monitoring becomes sensitive. In case an individual is tracked over a period of time, her movements and interactions can be analysed and behavioural patterns can be laid bare. Camera surveillance may reveal how an individual performs her work tasks as well as how she interacts with colleagues. These data reveal more than information about an individual's

---

[4] The Hygiene Guard® has primarily been developed for restaurant and hospital workers. It is for instance used in American casinos. See http://captology.stanford. edu/resources/cep/catalog/hg.html.

work activities. To a certain extent, values and beliefs are expressed in the way a person acts. The behaviour or habits exposed need not be socially stigmatising in order to be privacy sensitive. It can be socially acceptable but according to the individual, too embarrassing or private to share with others *e.g.* one's unstructured and haphazard ways of carrying out assigned work tasks.

A fourth subcategory is information concerning *personal belongings and private spaces at work.* There are certain spaces that employees consider private within the workplace, and they do have legitimate claims to privacy at work, especially in places where personal belongings are kept, such as cupboards or drawers. But privacy can also be expected in the midst of a work team, and concern one's workstation such as a particular desk/bench and certain work equipment. Social relations at work also belong to an employee's private space.

Furthermore, combinations of information can be privacy sensitive. Information that may be harmless *per se* can become privacy sensitive when combined with other data. The original purpose for obtaining the data may be obscured and the range and scope may be altered. We may have consented to each of *a*, *b*, and *c* but not to the sum of *a* + *b* + *c*. Within the workplace, information such as time, location and how work-tasks are carried out do in combination create a detailed image of the employee.

Purpose

The motives and reasons for implementing monitoring in the workplace are important for the way in which the technology is received and perceived. Personal information obtained can be used to improve work procedures and productivity *e.g.* by means of Electronic Performance Monitoring (EPM), and medical tests can serve to enhance safety. Under certain conditions EPM can provide an employee with a receipt of her good work, but it can also be used as a "whip." To exemplify the latter, Electronic Performance Monitoring has been used to identify an employee's maximum work capacity, only to raise the level once she achieved her maximum capacity (OTA report, 1987). Likewise, medical tests can be used to protect and further employees' health but also in ways that are socially stigmatising (EGE report, 2003).

Employees' views of workplace monitoring depend in part on whether they find the motive legitimate and the means reasonable, and whether they themselves benefit from the monitoring. In case the motive is insufficiently communicated or not accepted by the employees, they are likely to perceive monitoring as a sign of mistrust and as intrusive.

Monitoring is likely to be considered legitimate if it is used within reason (1), where there is a generally recognised and accepted need for a high degree of secrecy e.g. within competitive research or concerning national safety issues, or (2) to protect the health and safety of others, e.g. drug tests of pilots, taxi drivers and bus drivers, and possibly also (3) to evaluate work output. The utility that stems from monitoring and to *whom* it is beneficial is of great importance for how monitoring is perceived. In cases where we are under the impression that we benefit from surveillance in a substantial way, we are generally more benign to accept a certain degree of privacy intrusion. However, an employee need not achieve immediate personal gain as a result of monitoring. Rather, employees may be reasonable in the sense that they value "measure-ments" that imply a better work climate in general.

Three cases with different degrees of utility with respect to the moni-tored person will be presented in order to indicate how acceptance can be influenced by the way in which information is used.

In the first case, the individual benefits from the fact that she in par-ticular is being monitored, irrespective of whether others in a similar position also are subjected to monitoring. One example of this is the use of GPS in taxi cars. Taxi drivers are likely to accept GPS because of its security enhancing capacity even if the technology also enables tracing and tracking of the vehicle.[5] Likewise, even if biometric authentication within a company has certain drawbacks in terms of the employee being traceable,[6] the fact that the employee's work is facilitated in terms of quick and easy access to work stations and locked areas is likely to render her positive to this usage of biometrics.

In a second case, the person benefits from the fact that others are monitored in the same way as she is herself, and this gives her reason to accept that she, herself, is monitored. In this case, the principle of equity plays a significant role as well as reciprocity and mutual acceptance. The assumed security enhancement achieved through camera monitor-ing of public places makes a vast majority willing to accept limitations of privacy. Even though one, primarily, would prefer not to be subjected to monitoring, it might be considered acceptable due to (actual or ex-pected) positive effects stemming from monitoring.

---

[5] A MA-thesis at the Philosophy Unit of the Royal Institute of Technology, on the im-plementation of GPS in taxis in Stockholm 2004 indicated that most taxi drivers were positive towards GPS due to its safety enhancing capacity, despite its privacy inva-sive potential.

[6] The biometric information that enables authentication is often tied to a Radio Fre-quency ID (RF ID) making the individual employee traceable.

In the third case, monitoring is beneficial to others than the person who is subjected to monitoring. Single individuals may find it acceptable to be subjected to monitoring if for a good cause. A health care worker may accept the Hygiene Guard® system since hygiene and sanitation are of paramount importance in a hospital. A person with work tasks where good hygiene of less importance is more likely to find this kind of monitoring offensive.

A major purpose of analysing how information stemming from monitoring is used is to determine the distribution of benefits from monitoring. Three cases have distinguished between; 1) the monitored person benefits from being subject to monitoring herself, 2) the person benefits from general monitoring that includes the person herself, 3) the benefits from monitoring do not fall to the person who is subject to monitoring.

Surplus Information

Privacy intrusions do not necessarily occur as a result of an employer's actual usage of personal information about an employee. Certain surveillance capable technologies give rise to excess information and to a potential risk that such information (explicit or implicit) is revealed and used. In many cases, the data subject is unaware of the extra information collected, but for some "surveillance technologies" it is known that excess information is unavoidable. Within biometrics, the iris scan enjoys a reputation of credibility whereas the retinal scan, also measuring the eye, has given raise to privacy concerns since it reveals additional privacy sensitive information *e.g.* about a persons' health state.[8] Genetic tests provide indirect information about genetic traits of the tested person's relatives as in the case of recessively inherited (monogenic) diseases *e.g.* Huntington's disease. Employees with safety critical jobs, *e.g.*, air traffic-controllers, have been tested for Huntington's since even early symptoms such as loss of eye-tracking ability can be detrimental. In such a case, an employee's family may, implicitly, become entangled in the test and excess information may go against their interest not to know. If a daughter decides to test herself for Huntington's due to a history of the disease through her mother's side of the family, the test results would indicate whether or not her mother also has the disease – plausibly compromising the mother's desire not to know (Häyry and Tukala, 2001). Excess information also occurs in the case of drug tests. Apart from possible traces of drugs or alcohol, a lot of extra

---

[8] Cavoukian. A., "Biometrics and Policing: Comments from a Privacy Perspective," Information and Privacy Commissioner, Ontario, http://www.ipc.on.ca.

information about the employee can be extracted from blood or urine samples, *e.g.* information about diseases, ongoing medical treatment, or pregnancy.

It is important to ensure that the monitoring practice avoids the collection of surplus information as far as possible. (1) Excess information should not be collected if that can be avoided, *e.g.* if there are other ways of obtaining the information needed that do not give rise to excess information, (2) if collection of excess information cannot be avoided, one should if possible refrain from storing it, and (3), if it has to be stored in order to save other information that is collected, access to this information should be reduced as far as possible.

Storage

The need for protection concerning privacy sensitive information in public databases has been recognised in most Western countries where data protection laws state that personal information should be protected and that individuals have a right to know what data about them has been stored, and also a right to review and correct misinformation. Worker privacy is *e.g.* protected by the International Labour Organisation (ILO) Code of Practice on the protection of workers genetic personal data (ILO, 1997).

Even though storage is explicitly regulated, managers are now facing the possibility of obtaining new types of information for which no routines of storage have been established. Modern surveillance technology gives rise to novel types of information in the workplace setting, *e.g.* medical information about employees and unique identifiers like biometric samples. These types of information have previously been handled by medical staff, respectively the police. Furthermore, advances in computer technology have decreased the cost of storing information and increased the capacity of storage. There is no longer a need to get rid of old data because of lack of space, and there seem to be no limits for how long data can be kept (Nissenbaum, 1998:576). The lack of practical constraints on data storage may imply a risk that more data than necessary is stored. Since databases admit storage of huge amounts of data, clear and distinct plans for retention or disposal are not practically motivated in the same way as before. In particular, there is a risk that many different types of information are stored in such ways that privacy sensitive combinations can be retrieved. Despite the convenience with easily accessible and extensive databases, sensitive personal information should as far as possible be scattered and dispersed on several databases. As already emphasised, combinations of different types of data may give rise to privacy invasions.

When collecting data that may be classified as privacy sensitive, it is important to have a clear plan for how that information is to be stored and safeguarded, disclosed and disposed of. Due to the risk that more data than necessary is collected and stored, it is important to question whether information obtained really needs to be stored, especially in case the information is of a privacy sensitive character. An assessment ought to pay attention to whether information is stored or not, what kind of data is being stored (with respect to obviously privacy sensitive information and to the categories given in chapter 3.1), for how long time it is to be stored and if retention and disposal periods have been clearly defined.

Access

The development of computer technology has had a large impact on to whom information about individuals is accessible. Even if archives with personal files on citizens have been public in many countries, few people have utilised the material. Prior to computerisation and advanced networking capabilities, information was costly to achieve in terms of both time and effort. As acquisition and transmission of information have become inexpensive, a larger number of people have got access to personal data (Nissenbaum, 1998:577). Three aspects are significant for whether access to personal data is perceived of as intrusive or not.

Firstly, the number of persons with access to sensitive personal data is of importance with regards to privacy invasiveness. There is a difference if one single person or 1000 persons have access to one's personal information. This is not to say that the number of persons *implies* intrusiveness. Personal data in the hands of a large number of unknown persons may be perceived of as less problematic than the same information in the hands of a single person, but a person with whom one has a relation. However, given that all of those with access to privacy sensitive data lack personal relations with the data subject, she would most likely prefer having her information accessible to a smaller group of people than a larger.

Secondly, it is significant if those with access to personal data also have access to other types of data about the same person. Information that *per se* is perceived as harmless may become privacy sensitive in combination with or in relation to other types of information.

A third aspect of great import is whether the data possessor also can assert influence over the data subject. A traditional dilemma has been to what extent authorities should have access to personal information. Such information can in itself be a source of power. In a similar vein, the power imbalance between employer and employee can be reinforced by

169

the employer's access to personal information about an actual or prospective employee. This imbalance may stifle individuals' autonomy. Usually, we can choose what to reveal of ourselves, and to a certain extent, influence how others perceive us, but in the employer-employee relation, this ability is somewhat maimed. In the pre-employment context, a job applicant's weakness in comparison with the employer may result in a pressure to provide personal information required by the employer (EGE report, 2004). A pressure on actual or potential employees to state personal information is especially critical with regard to genetic information that may affect a person's access to opportunities and fair procedures.

Hence, it is important that the number of persons with access to privacy sensitive information about employees is limited as far as possible, especially those who also may assert influence or power over the data subject. Accessibility is foremost, but not exclusively a question of others' access to personal information about the data subject. Health surveillance and genetic testing may provide a person with information that she would have preferred not to have about herself.

Awareness

Personal information about employees can be obtained in various subtle ways by means of an invisible "control tower" *e.g.* by means of barely visible surveillance equipment. The degree to which employees are aware of workplace monitoring influences whether the practice is perceived of as privacy invasive or not. Information of the means and ends of monitoring is necessary in order for individuals to be able to protect their privacy. That is, we protect our privacy depending on what intrusions we anticipate. Since camera surveillance has become a normal part of the urban infrastructure, people calculate on the possibility of being seen by an invisible other and act accordingly, *i.e.* as they would feel comfortable being seen.[9] Conscious of the potential of being filmed in public people can choose whether to adjust their behaviour accordingly or not. Due to the public awareness of camera monitoring of squares and metros (and due to a seemingly general sympathy with the cause), this type of monitoring is seldom the target of accusations of serious privacy invasiveness.

---

[9] It is not necessarily the ability to adjust a behaviour one is certain of would find acceptance and liking in the eyes of others, but rather that of having a fair chance to choose to do so, that is of importance for privacy protection.

First and foremost, actual and potential employees need to know whether monitoring occurs within a company, that is, if they may become subjected to monitoring. For the prospective employee it is crucial to know if monitoring will at all be conducted.

Second, knowing that one may become subject to monitoring at the workplace, it is important to know the *kind* of monitoring one may be subjected to, *i.e.* whether it will be covert or overt, announced or random. It makes a significant difference in being aware that one may become subjected to monitoring even if one, at the time when the monitoring takes place, will not be aware thereof. Likewise, it is of importance if drug testing is pre-announced or conducted at random.

Third, it is important for employees to know the reasons *why* monitoring is conducted; whether monitoring is implemented to identify bottlenecks in production, to come to terms with employee theft, to enhance security *etc.*, but also if there is a norm or template against which their performance is evaluated. Privacy protection arguments drawing on control often imply an emphasis on the importance of a chance for individuals to adjust to socially acceptable standards or norms, and in this case, norms and customs that prevail within a firm. There is a significant difference if one adjusts to an explicit norm or well-known standard as in the case of the Hygiene Guard or if one adjusts to a standard assumed to prevail. Transparency concerning the reasons for monitoring and the underlying norms is preferable since that reduces uncertainty among employees. Uncertainty about the motives for monitoring may lead employees to unnecessarily impose demands on themselves that may cause stress and insecurity.

Influence

The way in which monitoring is perceived is coloured by the data subject's ability to influence whether and how she is monitored. Research on the effects of monitoring on workplaces indicates that in cases where managerial staff has communicated the reasons for introducing a monitoring system and employees have had the possibility to influence the implementation, they have, to a larger extent, focused on positive aspects of monitoring (Aiello and Kolb, 1995; Mason, 2001; Ottensmeyer and Heroux, 1991:522). Hence, it is of great importance that employees are represented (in the process) when monitoring device is being introduced in a company.

But even though employees are given the chance to raise demands on monitoring it is important to bear in mind that they are in a weak position *vis-à-vis* the employer when it comes to advocating their interests. Employees are typically in a weak position to influence whether they shall be monitored at all.

Control over personal data is usually exercised through informed consent, and this is frequently used as a criterion to determine whether monitoring is acceptable or not. To give one's informed consent to a practice is normally taken to mean that one voluntarily agrees without being pressured or coerced. However, a person who applies for a job where monitoring is conducted, has not necessarily freely consented to that practice. Many people accept certain disadvantages with a prospective job and prefer to work under conditions they do not fully approve of rather than not to work at all. Furthermore, even if the employee accepts monitoring from the beginning, this acceptance may come to change over time.

The work contract is normally preceded by interviews and tests, some of which require that the job applicant state personal information as in the case of drug and pregnancy testing. It could be argued that the applicant consents to give up this information, that she exercises her right to choose whether to accept testing or not despite potentially unpleasant consequences of a refusal to undertake a required test. But would that be a fair description of the individual's alternatives? She is to a large extent dependent on the prospective employer's acceptance and liking and it is virtually impossible for her to refuse, to withdraw or to modify consent without loosing the job offer. She has compelling reasons to give up the required information. Since informed consent is insufficient as privacy protection in the workplace, a possibility for employees to influence monitoring must be guaranteed.

In order for employees to be able to, in a free and informed manner, assert influence on the ways in which monitoring is conducted within a company they need to be informed about the whole implementation process, starting with (1) the company's reasons for implementing monitoring in the first place and (2) why monitoring is considered to be a reasonable means to achieve the aim, and (3) whether less intrusive means whereby the same ends could be achieved have been sought. The last point could concern the extent of monitoring, *i.e.*, whether there is good reasons for continuous rather than sporadic monitoring.

It has been emphasised that employees' so-called informed adjustment to monitoring is only in part a successful way of dealing with privacy intrusiveness. In the long run, adjustment is likely to be straining, especially if employees adopt a behaviour they are uncomfortable with. Unnecessarily privacy invasive effects of monitoring could be reduced by allowing for feedback from employees and ensuring the possibility of joint and continuous evaluation. When assessing a moni-

172

toring device or practice, consent should be treated cautiously. It is of great import to evaluate what possibilities employees have to abstain from the practice in question.

4. Conclusion

It has been argued that there are reasonable expectations on privacy in public and semi-public areas (such as the workplace) that ought to be recognised. Most surveillance practices are likely to, under certain conditions, constitute privacy invasions. While at times monitoring may be justified, restraints are required in order to safeguard employees' reasonable expectations on privacy in the workplace. Seven factors of importance for perceived privacy intrusiveness have been identified. The dimensional analysis is suggested as an instrument for assessing actual or potential monitoring devices and practices and the severity of privacy intrusions. It is proposed that by systematically trying to reduce the privacy intrusiveness of workplace monitoring in all these seven aspects, minimally intrusive means and ways of monitoring can be reached. Even if the negative effects of monitoring cannot be eliminated altogether, in most practical cases, the negative effects can be significantly reduced. Every reduction along one of these dimensions is to be considered an improvement.

References

Aiello, J. R., and Kolb, K. J., "Electronic Performance Monitoring and Social Context: Impact on Productivity and Stress," *Journal of Applied Psychology*, 80, 1995, 339-353.

Carson, S. A., "Drug Testing and Privacy: Why Contract Arguments Do Not Work," *Business and Professional Ethics Journal*, 14(4), 1995, 3-22.

Cavoukian, A., "Biometrics and Policing: Comments from a Privacy Perspective," Information and Privacy Commissioner, Ontario, available at: http://www.ipc.on.ca.

EGE (European Group on Ethics in Science and New Technologies to the European Commission), Opinion on the Ethical Aspects of Genetic Testing in the Workplace, Opinion No.18, 28th July, 2003.

Fried, C., "Privacy (A Moral Analysis)," in F. D Schoeman (ed.), *Philosophical Dimensions of Privacy: An Anthology*, Cambridge, Cambridge University Press, 1984.

Häyry, M. and Tukala, T., "Genetic Information, Rights, and Autonomy," *Theoretical Medicine*, 22, 2001, 403-414.

Inness, J. C., *Privacy, Intimacy and Isolation*, Oxford, Oxford University Press, 1992.

Mason, D., "Call Centre Employees' Responses to Electronic Monitoring: Some Research Findings," *Work, Employment and Society*, 15(3), 2001.

Marx, G. T., "Ethics for the New Surveillance," *The Information Society*, 14, 1998, 171-185.

Nissenbaum, H., "Protecting Privacy in an Information Age: The Problem of Privacy in Public," *Law and Philosophy*, 17, 1998, 559-596.

OTA. (Office of Technology Assessment), US Congress, "The Electronic Supervisor: New Technology, New Tensions," Washington, DC, 1987.

Ottensmeyer, E. J. and Heroux, M. A., "Ethics, Public Policy, and Managing Advanced Technologies: The Case of Electronic Surveillance," *Journal of Business Ethics*, 10, 1991, 519-526.

Persson, A. and Hansson SO., "Privacy at Work – Ethical Criteria," *Journal of Business Ethics*, 42, 2003, 59-70.

Rachels, J., "Why Privacy Is Important," *Philosophy and Public Affairs*, 4 (4), 1975, 323-333.

Regan, P.M. "Genetic Testing and Workplace Surveillance," in David Lyon and Elia Zureik (eds.), *Computers, Surveillance and Privacy*, Minneapolis, University of Minnesota Press, 1996.

Rosenberg, A., "Privacy as a Matter of Taste and Right," *Social Philosophy and Policy Foundation*, 2000, 68-90.

Scanlon, T., "Thomson on Privacy," *Philosophy and Public Affairs* 4 (4), 1975, 315-322.

Tavani, H., "KDD, Data Mining, and the Challenge for Normative Privacy," *Ethics and Information Technology*, 1, 1999, 265-273.

The ILO Code of Practice "Protection of Workers Personal Data," International Labour Organisation, Geneva, 1997.

Thomson, J. J., "The Right to Privacy," *Philosophy and Public Affairs*, 4(4), 1975, 295-314.

Tunick, M., "Privacy in the Face of New Technologies of Surveillance," *Public Affairs Quarterly*, 14, 2000.

Warren, S.D. and Brandeis, L.D., "The Right to Privacy," *Harvard Law Review*, 4, 1890, 193-220.

Westin, A., *Privacy and Freedom*, New York, Anathema Press, 1967.

Williams, B., *Shame and Necessity*, London, University of California Press Ltd, 1994.

Conclusion

Sven Ove HANSSON and Elin PALM

The purpose of this book, and of the preceding workshops, was to combine different kinds of knowledge and experience that can shed light on privacy issues on work places. We have connected the discourse on new forms of genetic and biotechnological monitoring of workers with that on computer-based surveillance and monitoring. Furthermore, we have applied insights and methods from moral philosophy to the resulting picture, and proposed tools for analysis and policy development. This integrative work is reported in the individual chapters. In this final comment we would like, as editors, to add a few reflections on what we have learnt in the process.

There are important differences between biomedical and ICT-based monitoring. As can be seen for instance in Simon Rogerson's and Mary Prior's chapter, extremely intrusive monitoring of employees' work behaviour is technically feasible in computerised work processes. In contrast, Gerard de Vries, Karel Van Damme and Marja Sorsa all emphasise the limited reliability of genetic screening. de Vries warns us that discrimination may follow from the mis- and overinterpretation of biological tests.

The ethical issues in biomedical monitoring are dealt with in medical ethics, the most well-developed area in applied ethics. Ethical issues in ICT-based monitoring are treated in the much newer and less stable area of computer ethics. Although there is, as pointed out by Colin Bennett, an emerging consensus on data protection principles, consensus is much less developed in this area than in biomedical ethics. There is also a large difference in terms of professional responsibilities. The medical professions have precise conditions of entry and exit, and well-established codes stating the ethical responsibilities of their members. In contrast, the development of corresponding principles for the responsibilities of ICT personnel is at a much earlier stage (as reported by Rogerson and Prior).

However, this does not necessarily make the ethical issues in biomedical monitoring easier to deal with than those in ICT-based monitoring. Health-related and biological information is often particularly

175

sensitive. As is pointed out in Hansson's chapter, non-genetic tests that are currently under development may very well provide more accurate information than genetic tests in sensitive personal issues. Perhaps most importantly, as Gerard de Vries shows in the first chapter, predictive and preventive medicine differ in radical ways from classical clinical medicine. Established ethical guidelines and principles that have been developed for clinical medicine may well turn out to be insufficient to deal with the new forms of medical practice.

The combined effects of biomedical and ICT-based monitoring have been at the focus in this work. In biometric identification systems, the two types of technologies are joined at the information creation stage. More importantly, if both biomedical and ICT-based information is available to one and the same person, then that person can combine them to create a more complete picture of the monitored individuals. As Elin Palm shows in her contributions, the privacy invasive effect of such combinations can be substantial, even if each individual piece of information is relatively innocuous. In Europe, such combinations of biomedical and ICT-based information are in most cases prevented by the ethical codes and the professional secrecy of the medical professions. However, this may be changed if employers demand such information from job applicants or if they receive it in their capacity as insurers, as many American companies do. It is against this background that Van Damme and Sorsa emphasise the need for a legislation that restricts the use of medical tests to what is in the patient's interest.

Several of the contributors emphasise the special nature of the workplace in relation to privacy protection. In important respects, the workplace belongs to the public sphere. As one example of this, pointed out in Hansson's chapter, an employer making a hiring decision is required not to discriminate. In his private sphere, for instance when he decides whom to invite for dinner, he is under no such requirement. As this example shows, to be an employer is, to some extent, a public office. But nevertheless, as Rogerson and Prior point out, we do have legitimate expectations of privacy on the workplace. These can be categorised as expectations of privacy in public. As noted by both Brey and Palm, privacy in public is a complex notion that needs careful analysis in order to be fully operative in a policy context.

Several contributors emphasise that rights to privacy at work have to be weighed against other legitimate interests, such as the employer's right to ensure that the work is performed as agreed and certain rights of third parties, such as that of passengers not to be driven by a drunk driver. Hence, a balance between interests has to be struck. Several tools are proposed in the book aim at facilitating the process of arriving at such a balance. Hence, Rogerson and Prior recommend the development of social impact analysis for this purpose. Persson proposes a procedure for determining when employees' rights to privacy are outweighed by the rights or interests of the employer or of third parties. For the cases when monitoring is defensible, Palm develops a dimensional analysis that can be used to identify minimally monitoring practices.

In the end, this is part of a more general issue, namely that of what an employer can require of an employee, and vice versa. In spite of the importance of work in our lives and in our societies, work-life has attracted very little interest from ethicists. Central issues in this area remain to be thoroughly investigated, including the moral implications of an employment contract, the mutual responsibilities of employer and employee, the moral distinction between work and non-work, and the special nature of workplace relations *etc.* These issues are made even more urgent by current changes in the organisation of work, such as the increased mobility at work (described in Bennett's chapter) and emerging new forms of contract where it is not so clear who is an employee and who is a business contractor. Privacy issues at work cut through most of these issues. The discussion of these issues can be seen as a probe for investigating workplace ethics. We hope that our use of this probe has shown that workplace ethics is a subject in need of much more scholarly attention than it has as yet received.

Contributors

Colin Bennett

Colin Bennett received his Bachelor's and Master's degrees from the University of Wales, and his Ph.D from the University of Illinois at Urbana-Champaign. Since 1986 he has taught in the Department of Political Science at the University of Victoria, where he is now Professor. From 1999-2000, he was a fellow of the Harvard Information Infrastructure Project, Kennedy School of Government, Harvard University. His research interests have focused on the comparative analysis of information privacy protection policies at the domestic and international levels. He has published extensively on privacy regulation. His most recent (co-authored) book is *The Governance of Privacy: Policy Instruments in Global Perspective* (2003). He was also co-author of a 1998 report for the European Commission on the methodology for assessing the adequacy of the level of privacy protection under Article 25 of the European Union's Data Protection Directive. He is currently involved in a three-year research project on the subject of privacy advocacy and activism.

Philip Brey

Philip Brey is an associate professor and vice chair of the Department of Philosophy, University of Twente, the Netherlands, and program director of the University's international master program in philosophy of technology. His research is focused on computer ethics and the social, cultural and epistemological roles of information and communication technology. He is co-editor (with Tom Misa and Andrew Feenberg) of *Modernity and Technology* (MIT Press, 2003) and member of the executive board of the international Society for Philosophy and Technology.

Karel Van Damme

Karel Van Damme is a scientific collaborator at the Centre for Human Genetics at the University of Leuven, Belgium. Van Damme is specialised in occupational medicine and been engaged in discussions on genetic screening. He has coordinated several European research projects related to socio-ethical and scientific aspects of genetic testing at work and other occupational health practices as well as several Bel-

179

gian inter-university epidemiological research projects in the domain of occupational and environmental health. Van Damme is also a fellow of the Collegium Ramazzini.

Sven Ove Hansson

Sven Ove Hansson is professor of Philosophy at the Royal Institute of Technology, Stockholm. He is also a member of the Swedish government's advisory board of researchers. He is editor-in-chief of the review *Theoria*. His research is currently focused on the philosophy of risk, value theory, and applied ethics. His most recent books are *Setting the Limit. Occupational Health Standards and the Limits of Science* (Oxford UP, 1998), *A Textbook of Belief Dynamics. Theory Change and Database Updating* (Kluwer, 1999), and *The Structures of Values and Norms* (Cambridge UP, 2001).

Elin Palm

Elin Palm received her MA in Applied Ethics from the University of Leuven, Belgium. She is currently a Ph.D student at the Philosophy Unit at the Royal Institute of Technology, Stockholm. Her field of research is applied ethics and her primary focus is on workplace adaptation of new technology and on establishing a model for Ethical Technology Assessment (eTA).

Anders J. Persson

Anders J. Persson is a Ph.D candidate at the Philosophy Unit of the Royal Institute of Technology. He is writing his thesis in connection to the research project "Ethical Problems in Work and Working Environment Contexts". His work belongs to the field of applied ethics with focus on work-related problems.

Mary Prior

Mary Prior is a Principal Lecturer in the School of Computing at De Montfort University, UK, where she is a Research Associate of the Centre for Computing and Social Responsibility. She has had extensive experience of undergraduate course design, delivery, assessment and management in the area of Computing and Information Systems in two higher education institutions in the UK. She is a member of the Institute for Learning and Teaching and the British Computer Society (BCS) and is a BCS examiner. She has worked for the Quality Assurance Agency as a subject specialist reviewer and for various UK universities as an external examiner. Her research includes an ongoing study of the ethical attitudes of Information Systems professionals for the Institute for the Management of Information Systems, and investigation of the ethical aspects of workplace surveillance. Publications include contributions to books, journals and conferences on these and related issues.

Simon Rogerson

Simon Rogerson is Director of the Centre for Computing and Social Responsibility at De Montfort University, UK and Europe's first Professor in Computer Ethics. Following a successful industrial career where he held managerial posts in the computer field, he now combines research, lecturing and consultancy in the management, organisational and ethical aspects of information and communication technologies. He has published widely and presented papers, many by invitation, throughout the world. His research focuses on technological assessment and qualitative stakeholder analysis. He has advised the European Commission on matters of ICT social policy and advised the Russian Government on the implications of the information society. He was a leading member on the Measures of Success project for the e-Envoy and the Implementation of Electronic Voting project as well as advising the government on the use of ICT to address social inclusion. He was the winner of the 1999 IFIP Namur Award for outstanding contribution to the creation of awareness of the social implications of information technology. In 2003 he was a finalist for the World Technology Award in ethics. He is a member of the Parliamentary IT Committee and Vice President of the Institute for the Management of Information Systems.

Marja Sorsa

Marja Sorsa is Director at the Department for Education and Science Policy at the Ministry of Education in Finland. Sorsa is docent in genetics at the University of Helsinki and former professor and research professor at the Finnish Institute of Occupational Health and the Academy of Finland. She is a member of the Bioethics Committee of the Nordic Council of Ministers, the Committee for Higher Education and Research (CC-HER), Council of Europe, the Working Party on Biotechnology (WPB), CSTP/OECD, the National Research Ethics Council of Finland and the European Group on Ethics in Science and New Technologies (EGE). She is also vice chair of the Board of the Finnish Genome Centre. Her list of publications includes c. 400 publications, of which about 250 in peer reviewed scientific journals and 140 presentations on international conferences.

Gerard de Vries

Gerard de Vries is Professor of Philosophy of Science and Technological Culture at the University of Amsterdam. An engineer and mathematician by training, Gerard de Vries turned for his PhD (1977) to philosophy of science. After a decade serving as Professor of Philosophy at Maastricht University and as Dean of the Netherlands Graduate School in Science, Technology and Modern Culture, de Vries joined the University of Amsterdam in 1997. He has published widely on philosophy of science, science studies, and particularly on the political, cultural and ethical aspects of science and medicine. His current research interests concern constitutional problems of risk societies, the politics of expertise, esp. in relation to risk-oriented medicine (genetics, epidemiology, health education) and relations between scientific knowledge, ethics and law.

Index

183

Tests, 11-12, 17-20, 28, 39-
52, 64, 74, 83-84, 102, 106,
114, 116, 119, 127-130, 137-
138, 148-152, 163
Global Information System
(GIS), 11, 162
Global Positioning System
(GPS), 13, 87-89, 166

H

Health surveillance, 11, 44
Huntington's disease, 19, 43,
167

I

Information and Communication
Technology (ICT), 12-13, 57-
58, 66, 68, 175-176
International Labour Organisation (ILO), 45, 50, 70, 82,
161, 168
Inequality, 13, 119
Information privacy, 13, 46, 70,
74-78, 80-85, 98, 101, 112-
113, 115, 119, 158
Informed
Consent, 23, 47, 49, 77, 83
Control, 99-104
Intrusion, privacy, 13-14, 90,
97-109, 112, 115-117, 119,
125, 132-133, 137-147, 150,
152-159, 160-173

L

Location-based surveillance
technology, 11, 64, 162, 164

M

Medicine
Classical, 21-22

Clinical, 12, 21-26, 28-29, 32
Occupational, 12
Predictive, 12, 17-21, 26-29,
32-33, 35, 39-42 29-50
Risk-oriented, 21, 27, 182
Mobile workers, 73, 86-92, 162,
164, 177
Monitoring
Biomedical, 162, 175
by camera, 166
Electronic, 11, 13, 47, 57-68,
70, 104, 110, 124, 165
Genetic, 40-42
of e-mail, 13, 60, 64, 83-84,
104, 110, 114-116, 137, 147
of software, 60-63, 74, 88,
108-109, 145-148
of the workplace, 59-71, 124,
138, 147-148, 157-158, 167

O

Occupational Health, 12, 17-18,
29, 40-52, 162-163
Office of Technology Assessment (OTA), 42, 124-125,
165

P

Predictive medicine, 12, 17-21,
25-36, 39-43, 128
Pre-employment tests, 40-43,
46, 160-161, 170
Pregnancy tests, 11, 32, 161,
163, 172
Prima facie right to privacy,
110-113, 139, 143-144, 146

"Work & Society"

The series "Work & Society" analyses the development of employment and social policies, as well as the strategies of the different social actors, both at national and European levels. It puts forward a multi-disciplinary approach – political, sociological, economic, legal and historical – in a bid for dialogue and complementarity.
The series is not confined to the social field *stricto sensu*, but also aims to illustrate the indirect social impacts of economic and monetary policies. It endeavours to clarify social developments, from a comparative and a historical perspective, thus portraying the process of convergence and divergence in the diverse national societal contexts. The manner in which European integration impacts on employment and social policies constitutes the backbone of the analyses.

Series Editor: Philippe POCHET, *Director of the Observatoire Social Européen (Brussels) and Digest Editor of the* Journal of European Social Policy.

Recent Titles

No.50 – *The Ethics of Workplace Privacy*, Sven Ove HANSSON & Elin PALM (eds.), SALTSA, 2005, 186 p., ISBN 90-5201-293-8.

No.49 – *The Open Method of Co-ordination in Action. The European Employment and Social Inclusion Strategies*, Jonathan ZEITLIN & Philippe POCHET (eds.) with Lars MAGNUSSON, SALTSA/Observatoire social européen, 2005, 511 p., ISBN 90-5201-280-6.

N° 48 – *Le Moment Delors. Les syndicats au cœur de l'Europe sociale*, Claude DIDRY & Arnaud MIAS, 2005, 349 p., ISBN 90-5201-274-1.

No.47 – *A European Social Citizenship? Preconditions for Future Policies from a Historical Perspective*, Lars MAGNUSSON & Bo STRÅTH (eds.), SALTSA, 2004, 361 p., ISBN 90-5201-269-5.

No.46 – *Restructuring Representation. The Merger Process and Trade Union Structural Development in Ten Countries*, Jeremy WADDINGTON (ed.), 2004, 414 p., ISBN 90-5201-253-9.

No.45 – *Labour and Employment Regulation in Europe*, Jens LIND, Herman KNUDSEN & Henning JØRGENSEN (eds.), SALTSA, 2004, 408 p., ISBN 90-5201-246-6.

N° 44 – *L'État social actif. Vers un changement de paradigme ?* (provisional title), Pascale VIELLE, Isabelle CASSIERS & Philippe POCHET (dir.), forthcoming, ISBN 90-5201-227-X.

No.43 – *Wage and Welfare. New Perspectives on Employment and Social Rights in Europe*, Bernadette CLASQUIN, Nathalie MONCEL, Mark HARVEY & Bernard FRIOT (eds.), 2004, 206 p., ISBN 90-5201-214-8.

No.42 – *Job Insecurity and Union Membership. European Unions in the Wake of Flexible Production*, M. SVERKE, J. HELLGREN, K. NÄSWELL, A. CHIRUMBOLO, H. DE WITTE & S. GOSLINGA (eds.), SALTSA, 2004, 202 p., ISBN 90-5201-202-4.

N° 41 – *L'aide au conditionnel. La contrepartie dans les mesures envers les personnes sans emploi en Europe et en Amérique du Nord*, Pascale DUFOUR, Gérard BOISMENU & Alain NOËL, 2003, en coéd. avec les PUM, 248 p., ISBN 90-5201-198-2.

N° 40 – *Protection sociale et fédéralisme*, Bruno THÉRET, 2002, en coéd. avec les PUM, 495 p., ISBN 90-5201-107-9.

No.39 – *The Impact of EU Law on Health Care Systems*, Martin MCKEE, Elias MOSSIALOS & Rita BAETEN (eds.), 2002, 314 p., ISBN 90-5201-106-0.

No.38 – *EU Law and the Social Character of Health Care*, Elias MOSSIALOS & Martin MCKEE, 2002, 259 p., ISBN 90-5201-110-9.

No.37 – *Wage Policy in the Eurozone*, Philippe POCHET (ed.), Observatoire social européen, 2002, 286 p., ISBN 90-5201-101-X.

N° 36 – *Politique salariale dans la zone euro*, Philippe POCHET (dir.), Observatoire social européen, 2002, 308 p., ISBN 90-5201-100-1.

No.35 – *Regulating Health and Safety Management in the European Union. A Study of the Dynamics of Change*, David WALTERS (ed.), SALTSA, 2002, 346 p., ISBN 90-5201-998-3.

No.34 – *Building Social Europe through the Open Method of Co-ordination*, Caroline DE LA PORTE & Philippe POCHET (eds.), SALTSA/Observatoire social européen, 2002, 311 p., ISBN 90-5201-984-3.

N° 33 – *Des marchés du travail équitables ?*, Christian BESSY, François EYMARD-DUVERNAY, Guillemette DE LARQUIER & Emmanuelle MARCHAL (dir.), Centre d'Études de l'Emploi, 2001, 308 p., ISBN 90-5201-960-6.

No.32 – *Trade Unions in Europe: Meeting the Challenge*, Deborah FOSTER & Peter SCOTT (eds.), 2003, 200 p., ISBN 90-5201-959-2.

No.31 – *Health and Safety in Small Enterprises. European Strategies for Managing Improvement*, David WALTERS, SALTSA, 2001, 404 p., ISBN 90-5201-952-5.

No.30 – *Europe – One Labour Market?*, Lars MAGNUSSON & Jan OTTOSSON (eds.), SALTSA, 2002, 306 p., ISBN 90-5201-949-5.

No.29 – *From the Werner Plan to the EMU. In Search of a Political Economy for Europe*, Lars MAGNUSSON & Bo STRÅTH (eds.), SALTSA, 2001, 526 p., ISBN 90-5201-948-7.

M. SVERKE, J. HELLGREN, K. NÄSWALL, A. CHIRUMBOLO,
H. DE WITTE & S. GOSLINGA

Job Insecurity and Union Membership
European Unions in the Wake of Flexible Production

In Europe, as well as in other industrialized economies all over the
world, employment relations have undergone profound transformations
over the last decades. Large numbers of workers have been displaced,
involuntarily employed part-time, or hired on temporary employment
contracts. The increasing flexibility in the staffing of organizations is
experienced, by many employees, as a threat to the continuation of their
employment relationships. A growing body of research suggests that
such job insecurity can be of fundamental importance from the
occupational health perspective as well as the managerial, due to its
effects on employees' work attitudes and well-being.

This book addresses the nature of job insecurity and investigates its
consequences for individuals, the organizations they work for, as well
as their labor unions. It also examines whether factors associated with
union membership help employees to cope with employment uncertainty. The book is based on a European project involving Belgium,
Italy, the Netherlands, and Sweden.

Both individuals and organizations alike are harmed by the increased insecurity that prevails in working life today. By identifying
and explaining those factors which result in job insecurity, and
examining how the experience affects individuals, organizations, and
unions, the authors wish expand the body of knowledge concerning job
insecurity. Such knowledge can lead to a greater focus on this phenomenon within working life, and result in greater effort being put into
understanding how preventative measures can be implemented in the
future.

Brussels, P.I.E.-Peter Lang, 90-5201-202-4, 2004, 202 p.

39.00 SFR   26.60 €*   24.90 €**   17.40 £   29.95 US$

* includes VAT – only valid for Germany and Austria – ** does not include VAT

Our prices are subject to change without notice.

DAVID WALTERS

Health and Safety in Small Enterprises
European Strategies for Managing Improvement

This book represents a unique contribution to discourse on protecting and promoting the health, safety and welfare of workers at a time of enormous change in the structure and organisation of work. It links regulating improvements in health and safety to structures and processes in the social and economic environment of small enterprises and in this respect provides an important departure from traditional analysis of health and safety regulation.

Its concentration on health and safety issues in small workplaces and peripheral forms of employment and its linkage of the means of regulating improvements in these areas to wider strategies for the reform of social and economic policies and practices in EU member states represent a serious attempt to contextualise both the problem and its solutions. Its focus on the role of diverse social and economic actors such as trade unions, large employers, insurance organisations, business support services and health care providers further illustrates the range and complexity of the subject.

David Walters is Professor of Occupational and Environmental Safety and Health at South Bank University, London.

Brussels, P.I.E.-Peter Lang, 90-5201-952-5, 2001, 404 p.
62.00 SFR   42.70 €*   39.90 €**   26.00 £   47.95 US$
* includes VAT – only valid for Germany and Austria – ** does not include VAT
Our prices are subject to change without notice.